This is a wonderfully empowering and educational read for anyone wanting to make positive changes to their breathing and their life.
Alison paints a truly holistic picture, full of clear and practical advice for the journey towards optimum health. Prepare to feel inspired.

Cheryl Mason MSc, BSc, BA, BSCH, MBAcC, PGCHE
Association of Chartered Physiotherapists Tutor

Alison blends her unique combination of knowledge and experience as an Osteopath, Hypnotherapist, Buteyko Breathing tutor and Naturopathic Specialist. The result is an integrated approach, promoting health and healing of the physical, mental and emotional dimensions of dysfunctional breathing, and the myriad of symptoms that manifest as a result.
She expertly walks the reader through every step of the journey and with online video classes to support, patients have the benefit of first-class, evidence-based strategies from one of the UK's leading experts in naturopathic medicine. Her work represents a truly holistic approach for anyone seeking to *Breathe with Ease*.

Janet Brindley
Buteyko Breathing Association Teacher Trainer

You may have had asthma or a breathing problem for a long time and believed that inhalers were the only answer. Think again. Alison Waring's *Breathe with Ease* challenges this view—recounting her personal experience of transforming her asthma using breathing exercises alongside holistic techniques to improve overall health. The first four parts of the book, *The Body, Emotions, Nutrition* and *The Mind* lay the foundations for the practice.
The final part, *The Breath*, includes details of the Buteyko Breathing Exercise programme and Alison's own innovative Dynamic Breath Release exercise.
If you want to help yourself to breathe more easily then this book will help to guide you on your personal journey.

Tanya Hunt
Naturopath and Metaphysical Healer

This excellent book will be greatly beneficial to anyone interested in their own physical or emotional health, not just asthmatics. It is comprehensive, clearly written and provides amazing insights into the interrelationship of emotion, lifestyle, health and disease. It is filled with practical advice and techniques for the reader to regain control over their health and wellbeing. The importance of breathing well for everyone is clear. This is a must read for anyone with breathing complaints of any nature who will flourish if they follow the invaluable advice given within this book, and also for those wanting to understand more about the complexities of health and disease.

Sarah Boswall Wheeler
Musculo-Skeletal Therapist

When I was teaching undergraduate Osteopathic students, I used to suggest they take a step back and look at the big picture. That is what Alison has done with her book, enabling the reader to have a holistic and sensible approach to promoting good health and respiratory function. It is written without too much jargon and is easy to follow, with practical advice for making lifestyle changes that are achievable and sustainable.

It's a useful addition for any family bookshelf,
not only for those with breathing difficulties

Debbie Pogson
EFT (Tapping) practitioner and hypnotherapist

Bringing together both her insight as a therapist and discoveries from her own personal journey to better health, Alison's book reveals the physiological, emotional and lifestyle factors which may be contributing to your condition. It offers a truly holistic approach, bringing understanding of how you can make practical healthy changes in your daily life which will support your body to heal naturally, reconnecting you to breathing and living with ease

BREATHE
WITH EASE

HOW TO ALLEVIATE ASTHMA AND TRANSFORM YOUR BREATHING HEALTH—
A NATURAL APPROACH

Alison Waring

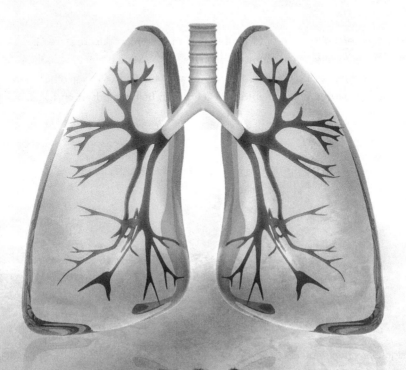

dot dot dot publishing

First Published in Great Britain 2018 by dot dot dot publishing
www.dotdotdotpublishing.com

This book is not intended as a substitute for the advice of qualified medical practitioners. The reader should regularly consult a doctor in matters relating to their health and particularly with respect to any symptoms that may require diagnosis or medical attention.

A catalogue record for this book is available from the British Library

ISBN—978-1-907282-88-1

Design by Martyn Pentecost ©2018 mPowr Limited
DotDotDot Logo ©2018 mPowr Limited

dot dot dot publishing

edge-of-your-seat books

To my dearest Thomas

You made completion of this book possible

Preface

Inspiration comes in many forms. None have been as powerful for me as seeing people transform their lives for the better. When I set out on my search for health, I had no idea where it would take me. The discoveries would not just help people overcome asthma, but would also help thousands on their path to improved health and well-being, finding the freedom to breathe with ease. Based on eighteen years of studying and practising alternative medicine, including osteopathy, guided meditation, naturopathy, hypnotherapy, Rebirthing and Buteyko, I have created healthier ways of living by truly embodying all I have learnt. I believe you too have an innate power and wisdom inside you that knows how to be well and healthy. In your hands is the key to your breakthrough. It is my desire to empower you to live life free from the fear of illness, stepping into your fullest health potential.

Having struggled with allergic asthma from the age of two until my early thirties, being able to snuggle up with a cat or stroke a dog without wheezing was something I never thought I'd be able to do. I had always loved animals, and they seemed to be attracted to me, but my body, and my lungs especially, didn't seem to like them very much at all. Was that really true?

At the time, I didn't know I had got lost in fear of animals from all the past reactions I had experienced. This only served to heighten the allergic response. If someone had told me there was something I was doing that was aggravating my situation, I wouldn't have believed them. At the time I felt that my body's reactions were outside of my control. It was just something that was happening to me. In this way, I fell victim to my body's internal reactions. I was fighting the constriction, as the airways narrowed, with my drive to breathe. To come to the point where you can work in harmony with your body, rather than fighting against it is liberating.

It is wonderful to now be able to feel a sense of stillness and ease inside myself around animals, which had long escaped me. If you can relate this experience to any situation which triggers a stress response inside of you, you can begin to sense the possibilities in your own life.

If anyone had suggested that I suffered from fear or anxiety, I would have replied, "Definitely not!" I had associated anxiety with symptoms of a panic attack, such as a fast-beating heart and sweaty palms and... *overbreathing*. When I finally understood how stress expressed itself in my body, and how it created asthmatic symptoms, I looked for ways to resolve the condition. Stress can present itself in many different ways in your body. There are two important areas to recognise and master; firstly, how do your body and breathing react during a stressful event, and secondly what happens with your breathing once a prolonged stressful event has ended? *Breathe with Ease* will guide you to mastering this as you begin to find ways to keep your breathing and body relaxed whatever the experience.

The idea that your body is self-healing is one of the fundamental principles of natural healing. Having been born into a family that trusted the body's innate healing ability, I had always wondered why the allergic asthma I had experienced since early childhood had remained and hadn't healed. That was until 2010 when I had a breakthrough experience. In three minutes I went from a full-blown allergic asthma attack to normal easy breathing, without medication. It was a moment of complete revelation to me to realise that I could work with my body rather than fight its reactions. *Dynamic Breath Release* was born.

If you have ever struggled with difficulty breathing and felt the panic of not being able to catch your breath, you will understand how completely out of control it can feel and how draining it is for every breath you take to be an effort. Would you like to be able to gain more control of your life and breathing, effortlessly? If you could achieve mastery with your body, emotions, thoughts and actions to create the life you have always dreamed of, what would that look or feel like?

Modern medicine doesn't provide all the answers. If you, like me, are passionate about natural health, rather than suppressing symptoms, you can work with your own innate intelligence to naturally enhance your health. It is not just breathing problems that can benefit. Breathing influences all aspects of your health. With *Breathe with Ease* and *Dynamic Breath Release,* you will discover how to work with your body, emotions and breath rather than against them. By letting go and working with your body to allow healing is incredibly powerful, you can learn to feel more in control than ever before.

If you would like to live your life naturally to the full, learning to breathe with ease through life's ups and downs is essential. This book will help guide you to master the many different aspects of life in relation to your breath. It will help you discover and clear the obstacles that stand in the way of your true health and well-being. The steps to mastery in this book are designed to show you how to make life-enhancing choices. Each chapter has bonus interactive elements; videos or guided meditations or exercises that complement your reading. Each section of the book is a signpost and stepping stone to your full health, enabling you to master breathing with ease.

Stepping Stones to Health

When we need to cross a river, we look for a bridge. Sometimes we have to make stepping stones to get to the other side of the river. Years before my breakthrough, I worked with a practitioner who was a bridge for me to experience that breathing with ease was possible. However, to be able to repeat the experience on my own and guide others through it, I had to place stepping stones in the river to get to the other side. This book outlines those steps so that you too can discover your full health potential and realise that it is perhaps easier than you think. Once the steps are in place, you too can be a bridge. This is your invitation to be able to breathe with ease...

CONTENTS

Introduction

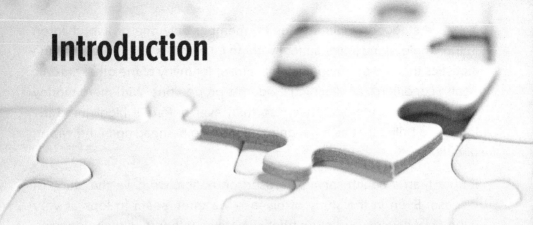

A journey of a thousand miles begins with a single step.

Lao Tzu

What do we all do around 20,000 times a day, often without even thinking about it? Just stop and pause for a minute and you'll soon be gasping.

Breathing.

Breathing is one of your most vital bodily functions. You can live without food for weeks, you can live without water for days but can live without air for mere minutes.

If you consider health improvement you might think about eating healthy food and drinking clean water, but how many people think about how they breathe? You may take it for granted that your breathing takes care of itself. With such a vital process is this wise? If you experience a struggle to breathe easily, with breathing difficulties such as asthma or shortness of breath, then breathing will be an issue that is at the forefront of your mind. However, many people don't even realise the importance of their breathing in relation to their experience of health and disease.

Focus on Health, not Disease

I was surprised to discover there were 5.4 million people with asthma[1] in the UK alone. One in eleven children are diagnosed with asthma.

This is a staggering increase as I remember only one or two children in the whole of my junior school with an inhaler. It is not just the asthma statistics that are this high, they are similar for many of the other chronic health conditions, all reaching epidemic proportions. With more money being spent on the health service than ever before, it highlighted my long-held belief that as a nation we appear to be heading in the wrong direction.

Rather than a health service focused on health, we have the study of disease. Even in the study of disease we often seem to look at very superficial causes, and often treat symptoms rather than the underlying problem. For example, with a bacterial infection destroying the bacteria without addressing why the internal environment enabled the bacteria to thrive is ill-advised. With chronic, long-term illnesses, we need to address the lifestyle habits that maintain the condition. Suppression of symptoms can, in the long run, lead to more chronic health conditions. It is good to know what causes disease, but we also need to realise what creates health.

What can Breathing Affect?

Effective breathing is highly important for people with breathing-related health conditions such as asthma and chronic obstructive pulmonary disease.[2] However, breathing patterns can also be affected in people with conditions ranging from anxiety and panic attack,[3,4] chest pain,[5] heart[6] and blood pressure problems[7,8,9] to diabetes[10,11] and thyroid disorders,[12,13,14] digestive disturbance,[15] headaches and migraine[16,17] and even types of epilepsy.[18] In fact, ineffective breathing and stress are inextricably linked. You don't have to be wheezing with an asthma attack to have ineffective breathing. You may just be breathing too much or too high up in your chest.

Although this book will focus mainly on the asthma and anxiety end of the breathing spectrum, many people have recovered their health through using the breath retraining and simple lifestyle changes highlighted in this book. If you have a medicated health condition, it is important that you work with a qualified practitioner rather than attempting to go through the exercises alone. If you are medicated for conditions such as an underactive thyroid, diabetes, heart problems or epilepsy, making lifestyle changes can affect the body's equilibrium. Being closely monitored is essential to have the correct support as you move towards health.

It is essential that any changes to whatever medication you are taking, even if it is for a breathing condition, be supervised by your doctor. It is important to have regular reviews of your medication, even more so if you are making lifestyle changes. Never stop steroid medication suddenly as this could prove fatal. Please continue taking your medication for any health condition until you see a doctor and only then make changes with their guidance.

How Breathing and Stress are Linked

If you have ever experienced the panic of trying to catch your breath and the exhausting effort that goes along with constricted airways or watched someone you love struggle to breathe, you will know how distressing this can be. Whatever condition you suffer from your ability to experience joy in life doesn't have to be limited. Transformation is possible.

When we become stressed our breathing rate increases. When our breathing rate increases it can also increase our experience of stress. Because most of the time your breathing happens automatically, these changes can occur without you being aware of them. As stress is a major contributing factor to many disease processes, then breathing effectively is one of the main keys to reducing your experience of stress and unlocking your full health and well-being.

As breathing is our most vital function, we seem to take it for granted that our body just takes care of it. We will explore the different factors which influence your breathing and how you can find a way to breathe with ease and naturally improve your health, energy levels and vitality.

Over time you have learnt ineffective habits of breathing which have been depleting your health. You can change this by retraining your breathing alongside some simple lifestyle choices.

Finding the Path

You will find out what hinders effective breathing, then you will learn practical steps that enable you not only to know how to breathe more easily but actually experience this. These are breathing techniques that will help transform your life, however, in order to gain the greatest benefit from them, you need to know all the areas that will help to support and strengthen your health along the way to create lasting change. There is no magic wand. In order to achieve lasting health, we must take a holistic approach. Focusing on one aspect of health can only bring half measures.

Even if you don't have a medical condition, *Breathe with Ease* can be used to achieve your peak performance, improve your concentration, immune system, reconnecting with your life force to give you a greater sense of wholeness.

There are many things that may stop you from breathing efficiently, and each chapter will address the challenges and then the practical steps to master them. The steps you can take have been broken up into five parts, the first four parts taking one week each for you to implement and the final section lasting four weeks. Which means that making the changes to enable good health becomes manageable and achievable for you, over an eight-week period. If you are feeling very enthusiastic, you can undertake the changes in weeks one to four in the first four parts of the book whilst doing the practice in Part Five over the same four weeks. You can take as long as you wish, there is no race. The most important thing to remember is that whatever you do sustainably will create more lasting change than doing something for a couple of weeks and forgetting about it. You need to build on the changes made in each section to establish good long-term health. If you have two parallel lines and change one by a fraction of a degree, eventually you will be miles away from where you began.

Although the book is split into five parts; Body, Emotion, Nutrition, Mind and Breath, each system is part of an integrated whole. Every section will address each system in relation to breathing and the other parts. For the best results, it is important to lay the foundations in the first four parts before you go on to the practice in Part Five.

Part One addresses *The Body*. This section will outline the basics of good breathing habits, some simple breathing anatomy (body structure) and physiology (body functioning) so that you can be aware of how and where to breathe to achieve good lung function. The causes of dis-ease and the fundamental principles of natural healing will be highlighted. It goes through exercises to improve the mobility in your thoracic cage and neck and how to prevent and reduce tension in your body with effective breathing.

Part Two focuses on *Emotions*. It will address how stress and emotions can affect your breathing rate and have health consequences. You will learn how you can reduce these through mindful awareness and bringing your attention to the present moment using the breath and positive affirmations to support your recovery. You will recognise how your fears and emotions can impact breathing behaviour and how to release them healthily with the breath. Breathing changes when you have different emotional states and you can change your emotional state through the breath.

Part Three gives you vital information about *Nutrition* and the common problems that can stop you breathing effectively. You will learn how to overcome excess mucus production, and abdominal bloating. You will discover which foods can affect your breathing patterns and your overall health and how to address food intolerances to reduce the levels of inflammation in your body. This section also looks at how you can overcome a health crisis naturally to bring you a greater sense of trust in your own healing ability, especially if you have been reliant on medication in the past.

Part Four looks at *The Mind*. One of the most important things I needed to learn in order for the breathing techniques to be most effective was hypnotherapy. The most successful clients I have seen for breath retraining understand how it feels to enter hypnosis and self-hypnotise.

You too can discover how to induce self-relaxation and enter this incredibly healing state in the interactive sections of this book. To process the large amounts of information we receive every day we often tune out in a state of hypnosis. This is a bit like having driven down the road in the car and suddenly realising you have been thinking about something else. We need to bring your breathing to the point where the breathing takes care of itself automatically *in a healthy way*. As you relax, so will your breathing.

In the final section, Part Five deals with *The Breath*; the bridge between your mind and body. You start to integrate what you have already learnt by carrying out a four-week breathing retraining session. If you are having an acute episode with your breathing, going straight to these methods first, after reading the first three chapters, will be of utmost importance. We can then deal with the lifestyle changes once your breathing has stabilised. If you are going through severe breathing difficulties, I recommend that you find a Buteyko practitioner who can work alongside you, with your medical support, to make sure you are on the right track.

Breathing is a behaviour, and just like any behaviour it can be retrained. As you learn the simple techniques, you will discover how easily and quickly it can change. Finally, you will bring together the understanding of how to integrate body, mind and spirit with the more advanced practice of Dynamic Breath Release. This comes from integrating my understanding of how to work with the body, emotion, mind and breath to transform your experience of health, bringing you the freedom to live your life to your fullest potential.

Note: All names in case studies or illustrations have been altered.

Further Free Resources Available for You Online

Breathe with Ease is accompanied by bonus online resources (videos, guided meditations, etc.) that supplement the information in each chapter. Revisit them as often as you need to support your practice. These *Steps to Mastery* will help you master breathing with ease.

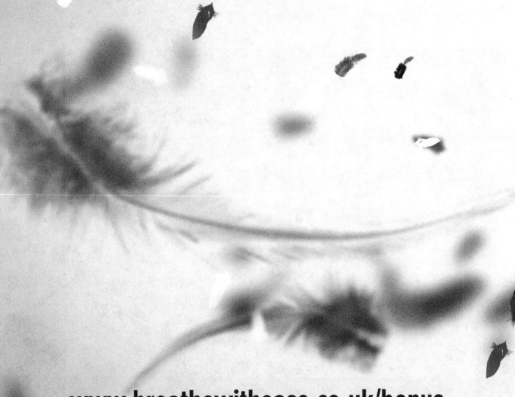

www.breathewithease.co.uk/bonus

If you wish to delve deeper into the research underpinning this book (linked to the superscript numbers throughout the text), download the reference guide.

www.breathewithease.co.uk/references

PART ONE—
THE BODY

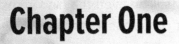

Chapter One

How Well Do You Breathe?

The nose is for breathing, the mouth is for eating.

Proverb

Paying Attention to the Breath

Just take a moment to experience your breathing. Without changing anything, see if you can notice how quickly you are breathing, and where your breathing movement is happening. Place one hand on your chest and one hand on your abdomen. Is the movement happening more in your chest or abdomen? Are you breathing through your nose or mouth? Is your nose blocked or clear? How many breaths do you take in a minute at rest? Time your breathing for one minute using a stopwatch and count your breaths. One breath includes an in- and out- breath.

How many breaths did you take? It is widely accepted that average normal breathing rate at rest in adults is around twelve breaths per minute. There are two parts to your breathing rate, both the number of breaths taken in a minute and the volume of the breath. At rest, we would ideally breathe around six breaths per minute.[19, 20] However, if they are six large-volume breaths you may still be overbreathing at rest. Your breathing can either be automatic or conscious, but thankfully we have mechanisms in place to keep us breathing even when we don't think about it. When we think about it, we might breathe more slowly or with more or less tension. When you don't pay attention to how you are breathing, old habits may creep in which can maintain dysfunctional breathing patterns which don't promote health.

Before you can improve your breathing, you need to be aware of what the bad breathing habits are, such as mouth breathing and upper chest breathing. As you check in with your breathing throughout the day, you can catch yourself and your breathing habits as they change during different activities and correct them. During different times of the day are you breathing through your mouth or correctly through your nose? Are you breathing high up around your collarbones and chest or, ideally into your abdomen?

Professor Buteyko, a Russian medical doctor, studied patient's breathing and discovered that people with chronic health problems breathed too much, known as hyperventilation or overbreathing.[21] By reducing both the rate and volume they breathed it made a significant difference to their condition, in many cases restoring health. Ideally, we would quietly nose breathe, using our diaphragm, with the movement occurring from our abdomen upwards. The average breathing rate is around twelve breaths per minute at rest; however, the Buteyko Method aims for closer to six breaths per minute. Slowing the breathing and using the diaphragm to breathe into your abdomen is one of the most important aspects of retraining your breathing.

Rapid breathing is linked to a stress or fight-or-flight response. You might not be feeling stressed mentally, but if your body is under stress, your breathing will increase and is likely to be higher in your chest; a typically asthmatic style of breathing, which also occurs with anxiety states. People with an asthmatic tendency have a lower threshold for switching from nose breathing to mouth breathing.[22] Asthmatic children also have a tendency to mouth breathe,[23] and adults with asthma typically breathe through their mouth when symptomatic.[24]

Mouth breathing for an hour each day has been shown to reduce lung function in mild asthmatics and initiate acute asthma symptoms in some.[25] Over time these habitual patterns of overbreathing can become the norm, throwing the body's systems out of balance. Switching to nose breathing and maintaining this is one of the first steps to master your breath.

So what causes you to breathe more rapidly and become a mouth breather in certain circumstances? Trying to breathe harder against resistance in the chest is one reason for switching to mouth breathing. Sometimes it is simply having a congested nose, or small nostrils or having had a nose injury. When we are born, we are designed to nose breathe so that we can feed and breathe simultaneously. Think about the sharp inhalation or gasp you take through your mouth if you have a shock. This primitive startle or stress response could become the predisposition if you have experienced a prolonged episode of stress. When you breathe in, there is an increase in tension in your body. As you breathe out all the muscles in the body can relax. However, if you become stuck in this pattern of inspiration without fully letting go on the out-breath, your body will retain a lot of tension, which will signal to the adrenal glands that there is a continuing threat, causing them to work harder. Eventually, the body becomes tired and it is often in the exhaustive phase that symptoms of breathlessness are usually experienced.

The Difference Between Triggers and Causes

It is useful to look at health from a different perspective. We often assume that the triggers of asthma are the cause, such as animal dander, dust or pollen, exercise and sport, cold air and infection. However, what if the trigger isn't actually the underlying cause? Knowing your triggers doesn't always help you to improve your health in the long-term, it could just lead to avoidance behaviour, which can be sensible but not always achievable. However, what if your triggers aren't actually the cause of the asthma? Finding the cause of why you react to the dust, animal dander or cold is what we need to understand in order to start making sense of how your body functions to help improve your health. Why do the lungs react and inflame to these triggers and how can you reduce the reaction?

Symptoms of most illnesses come about when we have a long-term stress response which may have started early on in life. The adrenal glands produce the hormones adrenaline and cortisol in response to stress. These open the airways and enable a fight-or-flight response so that we can get enough oxygen to deal with the threat and run to safety. Once the fight-or-flight response is triggered, an increased breathing rate will maintain the stress response, which is likely to cause hyperventilation if you are stressed and sedentary.

The stress hormone cortisol is a natural anti-inflammatory in your body. When you have enough cortisol, your body will work well. When your system becomes exhausted from long-term stress there will be a depletion in adrenaline and cortisol, which is why the medication provided for asthma treatment mimics adrenaline, in the reliever inhalers, to open the airways a cortisol-like steroid is used as a preventer to reduce the inflammation, so the airways remain open. This would point towards the asthma attack being a condition of adrenal exhaustion.

Prolonged stress reduces the function of the eliminatory organs, digestive system, and immune system as these are not of primary importance when dealing with an immediate life and death situation. Long-term stress can eventually lead to an exhaustion of the fight-or-flight mechanisms in your body, affecting many systems. The initial compensation of an increased fight-or-flight response will eventually lead to long-term adaptation which presents itself as symptoms of diseases, which is the body's survival strategy.

What caused your system to be overloaded? Some of the stressors may be things that you can change in your current life; some of them may have been programmed from a young age and may require some deeper work to resolve. Other stressful events, which may have created physical tension in your body, may have long gone, but we can still carry the retained tension from these emotional incidents. Another cause for the physical reaction of tensing is re-experiencing stressors similar to those of an initial trauma because the body tenses in an attempt to protect us. You may have noticed the flinching reaction you experience if you see someone hurt themselves. This reaction creates a protective armour around you, especially in the shoulders and ribcage and if you stay tense, muscles maintain their contraction and over time the body loses its flexibility and breathing can become more laboured.

By discovering the causes of your long-term stress that overloaded your adrenals and how to listen to your body more effectively you can soften your body and let go of the tension, experiencing a new level of relaxation. Rather than avoiding the triggers or overstimulating your body with medication, the easiest way to reduce the reactivity in your body is by slowing your breathing to reduce the background level of stress.

The Early Life Stressors and Your Set Point

There can be many causes of stress when we are an infant. If you had breathing difficulties in your early life, then early stressful events and crucially the way your body responded to those stresses may have been the cause of your health challenges. It is common to both tense your body and breathe more rapidly during these times. This can be a cause of symptoms at any age if your system becomes overloaded. The symptoms are simply the body trying to correct the imbalances that are created.

It is worth reflecting on where your breathing difficulties first started. For some people, it might start in early infancy, following a traumatic birth, a congested nose, a bereavement or reaction to an animal or food. For others, it might be during a stressful period in childhood or in adulthood due to cold weather, overexertion with sport or illness. These experiences may have been the tipping point of an underlying level of stress and physical tension that has built in the body over years and a habitual pattern of holding unconscious tension in your neck, chest, diaphragm or stomach. This could even have been learnt from our parents as babies. Young children will often pick up on the tension in their parents and have similar muscle tension patterns.

It is incredible to think that your earliest childhood experiences can create a set point for your background level of stress that stays with you through life, until you become mindful of your reactions. This means that even when we think we are relaxed there is a certain level of nervous tension in the body that is running without us being aware of it, causing a level of hidden hyperventilation. You can become aware of this tension in your body and be mindful of how you may tense different areas of your body in relation to stressful events. Do this by regularly scanning your body and relaxing any areas of holding. With practice and by including the breathing exercises you can begin to create a new, more relaxed set point in your body.

Having health challenges can have its benefits. It can give you direction and a sense of purpose that informs your life path, as it can create a desire within you to make a difference. If you have experienced suffering, you are more likely to be compassionate with others who have suffered too. Your sensitivities can be an asset to you if you learn to use them wisely. However, you also need to make sure that you take good care of yourself.

By taking the medication, we are simply keeping the body overstimulated to get through it, which in the long run can cause further problems. This may be a necessary lifeboat. Your body can become quite dependent on steroid medication in particular. Steroids should never be stopped suddenly as it can be life-threatening.

Breathing retraining has been shown to reduce the need for medication,[26] but you will need to practise the breathing exercises in Part Five consistently for at least four weeks to enable the possibility of medication changes under the supervision of your doctor. You need to build your health first. It may take six to twelve months to stabilise your health, integrate and maintain all the changes necessary, depending on the severity of your condition.

What Happens During an Attack?

When symptoms of exhaustion occur, the main tubes, known as the bronchi, which go to each lung, can start to constrict and increased mucus production can leave it difficult to exhale and relax. The expiratory wheeze, which is diagnostic of asthma, is often associated with a cough or nasal congestion and chest tension.

However, rather than feeling that your body is doing something unsupportive and not trusting your body, maybe the reactions are your body's way of trying to protect you. Buteyko believed that the reactions happened in the lungs as a way of trying to slow down the overbreathing and maintain the correct balance within your systems. Rather than overriding the symptoms your body expresses, it is important to learn how to work with your body, rather than fight it. Breathing bigger breaths when the chest feels tight will only exaggerate the problem. Breathing slowly and reducing tension in your body by relaxing your shoulders and breathing into your abdomen will begin to reduce the stress on your system.

A tickly cough or need to clear the mucus can become a habitual reflex reaction that can actually continue the irritation and dysregulated breathing. The more we cough, the more we maintain the airway inflammation. Unless you have something large to cough up, instead of coughing, try to repeatedly swallow two or more times and relax the space just below your ribcage. This helps the mucus to drain away and the diaphragm to relax. Coughing with your mouth closed can help prevent overbreathing. Coughing at night is also worsened if you experience post nasal drip which irritates the throat. By sleeping on your side, rather than your back, you can help to alleviate this irritation.

Similarly with the nose, the more you blow your nose, the more it can maintain the mucous membrane irritation, overproducing mucus, which can keep it blocked. You can measure your progress through your *Control Pause*. Having taken a normal-sized in-breath your control pause, or CP, is the length of time you can comfortably pause your breath from the end of your out-breath to your next in-breath. You must be able to regain your relaxed breathing immediately. Where in your body do you have to relax in order to lengthen this pause?

Caution: You should not attempt the full set of Buteyko exercises if you have any of the conditions listed. Keep your breathing slow and relaxed without the pauses, unless you are supervised by a practitioner.

STEPS TO MASTERY—Nose Breathing and Control Pause

Practise your quiet nose breathing into your abdomen for ten minutes twice each day. You can do this first thing on waking and before going to sleep. Your understanding of abdominal breathing and relaxed breathing will be enhanced by reading chapters two and three. You can check your control pause time (CP) before and after your breathing relaxation. If your breathing is really giving you challenges, skip straight to Part Five to go through the full breathing retraining process... and if you are having significant challenges and your control pause time is less than ten seconds, find a Buteyko practitioner who can guide you through the process.

Caution

In case you missed it... steroid use should *never* be discontinued without medical supervision, as the body can become dependent on the medication. Gradual reduction under medical supervision is advisable only once health has been improved significantly and new lifestyle changes have been adopted as a way of life. Your control pause time must be at least 25-30 seconds before seeing your doctor for a medication review.

When doing the control pause, don't push it too long, you need to be able to recover your relaxed breathing immediately, without taking a deeper breath.

If you struggle to clear your nose, you may need to spend a couple of weeks on a diet that supports a reduction in inflammation and mucus production.

People with the following medical conditions must *never* apply Buteyko without first consulting a doctor and an experienced Buteyko practitioner:

- Arterial aneurysm
- Haemorrhagic stroke
- Thrombosis
- Current cancer treatment
- Recent heart attack within twelve weeks
- Brain tumour
- Uncontrolled hypertension (high blood pressure)
- History of serious cardiac rhythm disorder (unless pacemaker fitted)
- Severe renal failure (includes dialysis)
- Uncontrolled hyperthyroidism
- Sickle cell disease
- Acute schizophrenia
- Chronic Obstructive Pulmonary Disease (COPD) with cor pulmonale
- Pregnancy (first trimester)

In some cases, a very mild therapy may be possible. People with the following conditions must take caution when applying the Buteyko Method. Again, always seek help from an experienced Buteyko practitioner, rather than using self-help learning tools.

- Diabetes, especially insulin controlled
- Mild/controlled hypertension
- Thyroid disease
- Angina/previous heart attack
- Epilepsy
- Past history of schizophrenia
- Reduced kidney function
- Pregnancy (second and third trimester)

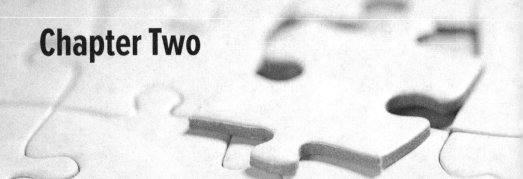

Chapter Two

The Structure and Function of Breathing

The noblest pleasure is the joy of understanding.

Leonardo da Vinci

Looking After Your Body

Breathing around 20,000 times a day into the upper chest causes considerable tension to build in the neck and shoulders. These muscles were not designed for continual breathing movement. Over time your body will intelligently lay down fibres within the muscles to hold them in a shortened state to lift the chest and reduce the energy required to contract the muscles used with upper chest breathing. This can produce aching and stiffness around the neck and shoulders as the blood flow into the muscles is reduced by the tension and a build-up of acid waste products can occur, further exacerbating the tension. With the correct diaphragm breathing, you can help prevent the build-up of neck and shoulder tension.

You may have found yourself putting your hands on your hips if your breathing has been laboured, especially after exertion. This automatically lifts the upper ribs and enables easier diaphragm breathing. Placing your hands on either side of your lower ribs, and dropping your shoulders, can you feel movement in your lower ribcage and abdomen as you breathe? You can either breathe into your sides or your tummy to improve your diaphragm movement. If it feels tight, you can use the exercises at the end of this chapter to improve your diaphragm breathing.

In order to breathe efficiently, it is important to know more about the structures involved in your breathing, how it works and how to release the tension in your body to enable easier breathing. One of the main principles of healing is that every organ and tissue requires a good blood supply for oxygenation and health to exist. We are going to take a look at how this actually happens.

Breathing Structure and Function

Your breathing occurs from an incredible dynamic interplay between the air surrounding you and the fluid, nerves and structure of your body in relation to your activity, be it mental, emotional or physical. Understanding body anatomy or structure provides a framework to understand how your body functions. Your respiratory system is protected by the thoracic cage, formed by the ribcage, which attaches to the thoracic spine at the back.

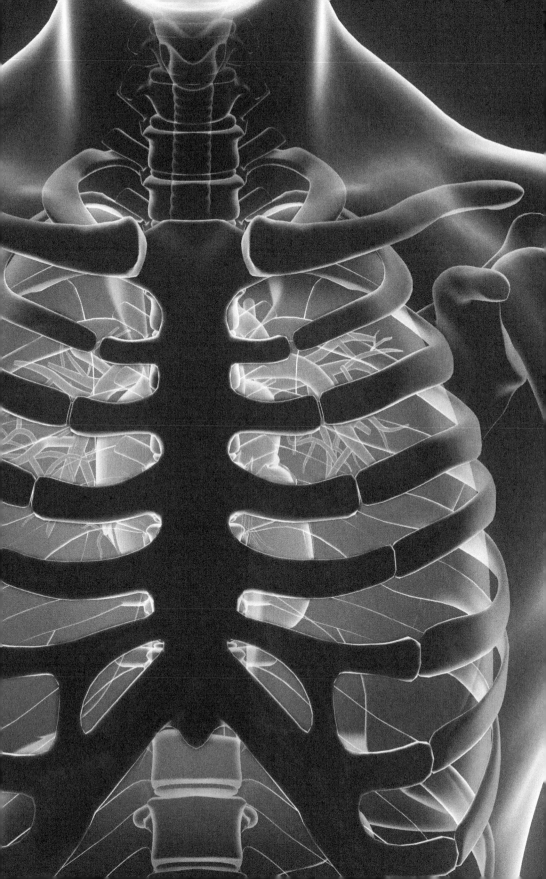

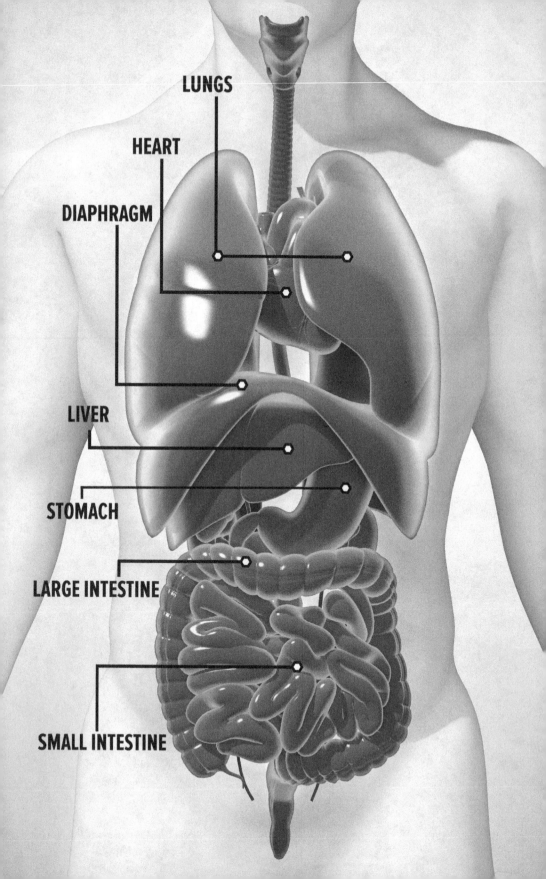

LUNGS

HEART

DIAPHRAGM

LIVER

STOMACH

LARGE INTESTINE

SMALL INTESTINE

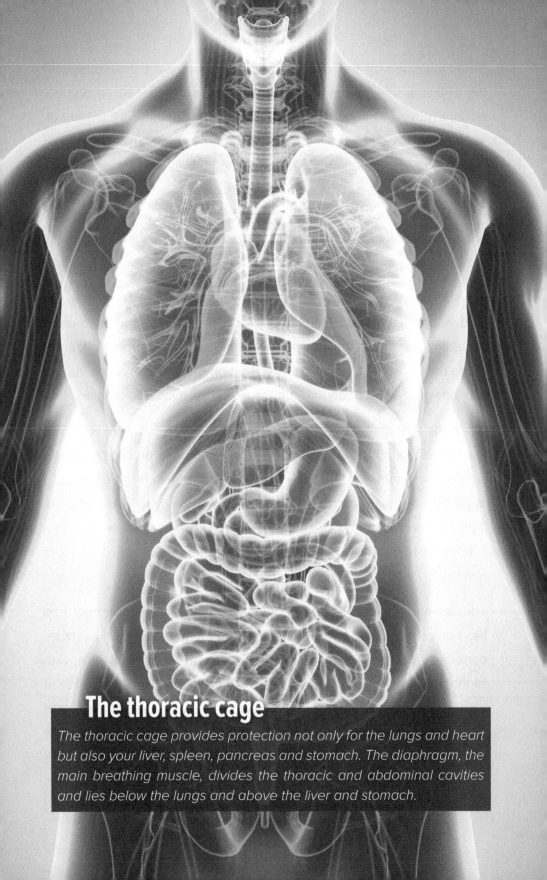

The thoracic cage

The thoracic cage provides protection not only for the lungs and heart but also your liver, spleen, pancreas and stomach. The diaphragm, the main breathing muscle, divides the thoracic and abdominal cavities and lies below the lungs and above the liver and stomach.

Breathing involves the expansion and relaxation of the ribcage as the breastbone (sternum) raises forwards and the ribs lift up and out on inhalation and lower on exhalation. As you breathe in, the sheet-like muscular dome of the diaphragm contracts, flattens and pushes down, expanding the lungs and massaging the internal organs below. As we breathe out, it relaxes back into its dome-like shape. This action also helps to draw blood back to the heart, similar to a sink plunger unblocking a drain, and massages all the organs below the diaphragm, including your intestines.

Breathing into your upper chest, there can be more congestion and stagnation of the deoxygenated blood in the abdominal organs. Breathing into the abdomen over time can help improve your abdominal organ health as it helps improve oxygenation of your internal organs and can aid waste elimination through the bowel, as it massages them.

When the airways become constricted the muscles between your ribs, known as the intercostal muscles, have to work harder and can often feel tight and resistant with breathing difficulties and there can be a tendency to breathe harder against the resistance. As you may have discovered, fighting this tension by breathing harder only makes it worse. At rest it is possible to breathe only using the diaphragm, allowing your chest to relax.

The saying, "breathe in," as people squeeze through a narrow gap has confused many people to their natural breathing movement. More correctly it is the abdominal muscles which are being pulled in, with slight tensing of the edges of the diaphragm, whilst you will notice your chest actually expands. However, it is really important to state that *as you breathe in your tummy should gently move out*. This is the natural breathing movement. Breathing out is a simple relaxation of this movement, unless we are exerting ourselves with exercise, or forcing an out-breath.

Natural breath movement

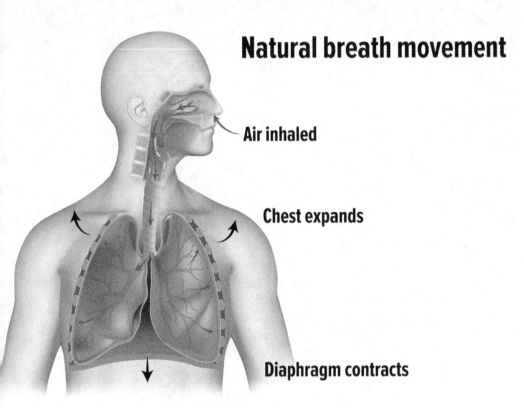

Air inhaled

Chest expands

Diaphragm contracts

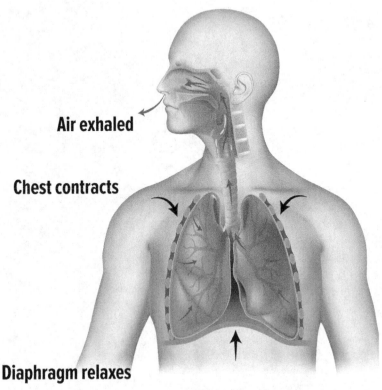

Air exhaled

Chest contracts

Diaphragm relaxes

To help you with diaphragm breathing, place one hand on your chest and one on your tummy and see if you can allow the lower hand only to move as your belly rises and falls. Imagine inflating a balloon of air in your abdomen. You can imagine breathing in and out of your navel if it helps. See if you can enable the breathing movement to happen from the bottom upwards, as though you were filling a glass with water. In this way, if you need to take deeper breaths during exercise, you are starting with the diaphragm before the ribcage rises. It should feel like a wave of movement from your abdomen upwards and then a retreat of the wave, from the top down, on your out-breath.

In many people, especially if you suck in your stomach, the majority of breathing movement happens just in the upper chest. To begin with, lying on your back with your head supported, relax your tummy muscles. Allow your tummy to gently rise and fall with your breath, which will engage your diaphragm.

Understanding Lung Function (Physiology)

When you breathe in, air comes in through your nose and circulates between turbinate bones which spiral the air, helping to warm, moisten and filter it, throwing any particles into the hairs and mucous membranes on the inside of the nose. As the air continues down through your windpipe (trachea), just below your neck the trachea branches into the two bronchi, which then subdivide into bronchioles and terminate in small grape-like sacs called alveoli. It is here where the exchange of oxygen and carbon dioxide occurs.

Lung structure

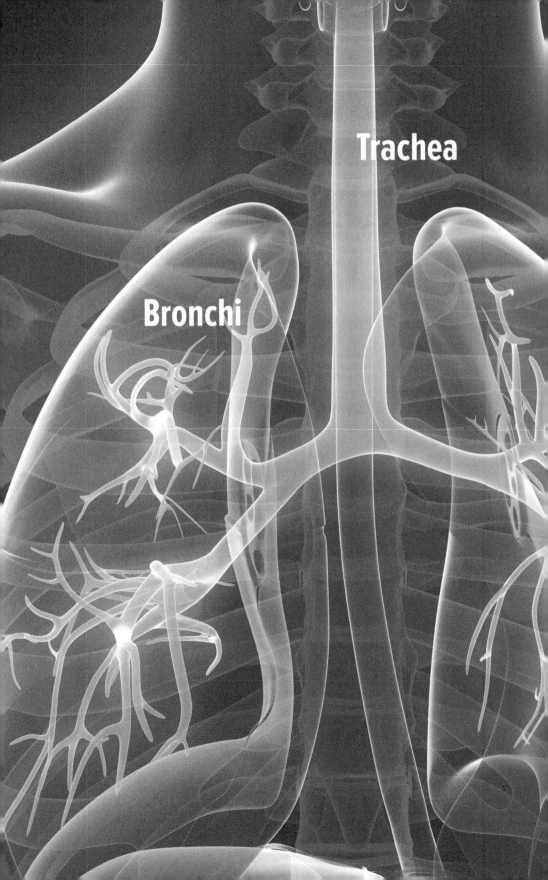

The lungs have around one-and-a-half thousand miles of airways and around three hundred to five hundred million alveoli. If the whole surface area of the lungs was laid out, it would cover seventy square metres, around the size of one side of a tennis court. It is amazing to think that there is only a single-cell thickness between the air coming into the alveoli and the tiny capillaries running next to these air sacs carrying the blood. The carbon dioxide diffuses out of the blood into the lungs and the oxygen diffuses from the lungs into the blood. There is a continuous flow of both gases in the direction from high concentration to low concentration.

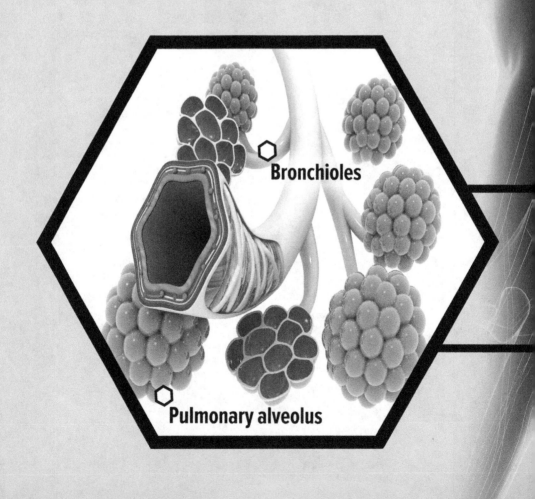

Bronchioles

Pulmonary alveolus

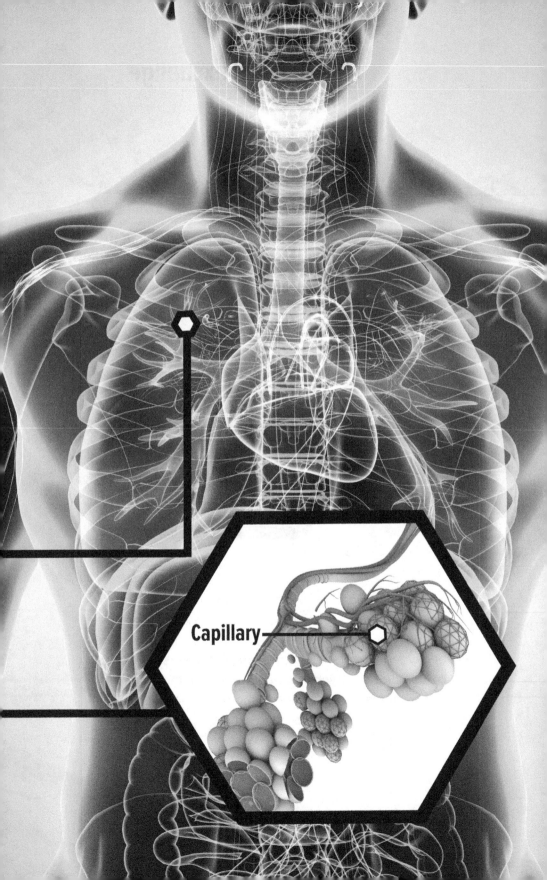

Capillary

Alveolus gas exchange

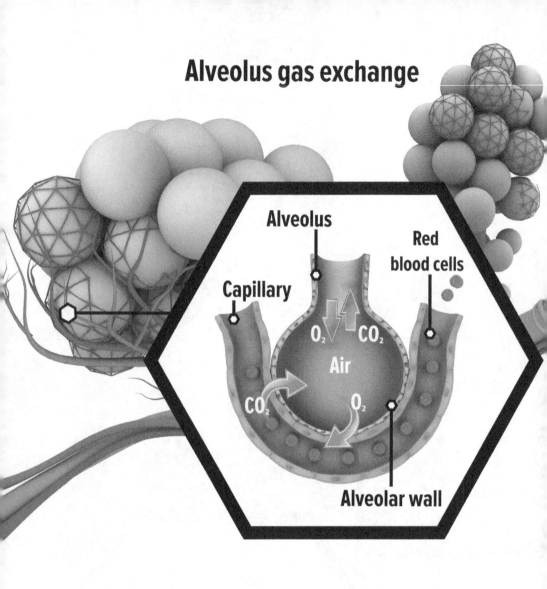

Alveolus

Red blood cells

Capillary

O_2 CO_2

Air

CO_2 O_2

Alveolar wall

Because oxygen has been used up in the body, when the blood returns to the lungs, there is less oxygen in the blood than from the air breathed in, so the movement of oxygen goes from air to blood. The reverse is true of carbon dioxide which is normally higher in the blood as it arrives at the lungs. The carbon dioxide moves from the blood into the lungs, which we exhale.

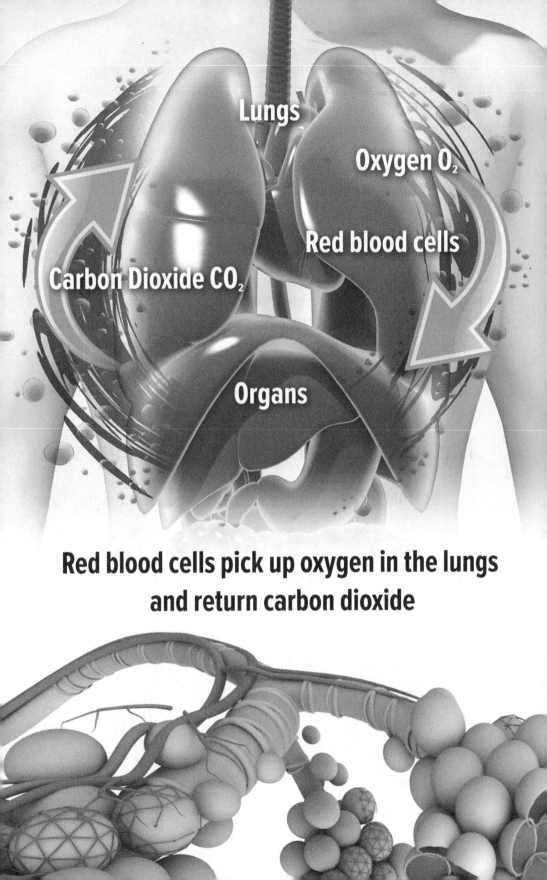

Red blood cells pick up oxygen in the lungs and return carbon dioxide

The red blood cells contain haemoglobin which carries oxygen and carbon dioxide gases in our blood. The haemoglobin lets go of oxygen where there are higher levels of carbon dioxide in our body, and picks up the carbon dioxide, taking it back to the lungs. It is, therefore, the carbon dioxide levels which trigger your breathing rate and the release of oxygen into your tissues. The more activity you do, the greater the volume of CO_2 being produced and the faster the breathing.

There are microscopic *hairs* known as *cilia* on the cells lining the passageways into the lungs, which help to waft the mucus up and out of the lungs. These cilia, known as the mucus escalator, are damaged by smoking. A cough may take a long time to clear because all seventy square metres may have to be cleared of mucus, all against gravity. If you have a cough that lasts longer than three weeks, then it is vital you see your healthcare provider.

When the lungs become inflamed during an asthmatic episode the bronchi narrow and there is an increase in mucus production which slows the movement of air in and out of the lungs, as shown below.

The airways in a normal and inflamed state

Normal Airway   During Asthma Symptoms

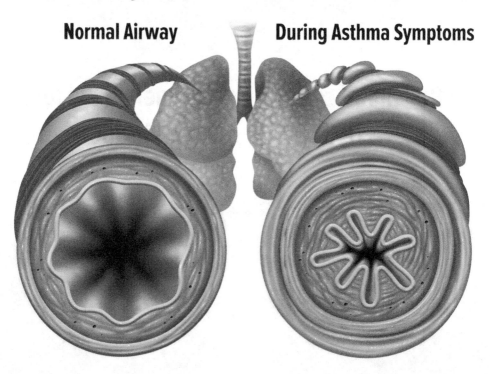

If you assume that the body always uses its tissue intelligence in whatever reaction it creates, one possible reason for this response is to slow down the hyperventilation or overbreathing, which if left to continue unabated would throw the blood biochemistry further out of balance and alter important chemical reactions in our systems. It forces you to stop and rest.

Cellular Respiration

The oxygen in the air that you breathe is used by all the cells in your body. Cell activity is fuelled by glucose joining with oxygen to form energy for muscle movement or other cell functions within the internal organs. This process is known as cellular respiration and creates carbon dioxide and water which you exhale from your lungs. When you exercise you will produce more carbon dioxide (CO_2) and more oxygen is required for cell activity. You will breathe faster to blow out the increased levels of CO_2. However, there is an optimal breathing rate that will enable the most effective oxygenation. As oxygen is released in the presence of CO_2, then by slowing the breathing rate so that our carbon dioxide levels can rise a little, more oxygen will be released into the tissues.

Physical activity creates a demand for oxygen. If the demand exceeds supply, the muscles can keep working for a period of time without oxygen. This process is known as anaerobic respiration. Carbon dioxide can be used instead of oxygen to create energy, but this forms lactic acid as a waste product, causing the familiar stitch feeling you will have undoubtedly experienced. The acid in the tissues creates pain. We breathe more rapidly during exercise not only to bring in more oxygen, but also to breathe out the acidic carbon dioxide. It is vital we keep our blood at the right acid-alkali balance for all our cellular reactions to function normally. If you have developed a habit of breathing too much at rest the acid-alkali balance will be tipped in the wrong direction leading to symptoms of hyperventilation, such as anxiety and panic, pins and needles, dizziness or light-headedness, visual disturbance, chest tightness, difficulty breathing, abdominal bloating, and a dry mouth and throat.[27]

Nerve Supply to the Lungs and Diaphragm

The diaphragm receives its impulse to rhythmically contract and relax for breathing from the phrenic nerve, which arises from between the middle three vertebrae on either side of the neck. This is because when you were an embryo, your diaphragm started in your neck and descended down to your lower thorax, taking its nerve supply with it. Mostly your organs have a nerve supply from the spine at roughly the same level as the organ position in the body. With the lungs, they have a nerve supply arising from the base of the skull and the upper back, between the shoulder blades. Making sure these areas are relaxed will help breathing function and nerve signals.

Structure and Function are Interrelated

Referred pain can occur in the spinal muscles when the internal organ becomes inflamed and sends an irritated signal through the nerves and back to the spine, and then the muscles supplied from that spinal level become irritated and tense. Because the skeletal muscles have more pain receptors than the internal organs, we can use this as an early warning system; you can often feel tenderness in the muscles related to an organ before any overt organ symptoms present themselves. This is an example of your body structure and organ function being interrelated. Similarly, you could have mechanical tension between your shoulder blades that would irritate the nerves to the lungs and make the lungs more sensitive and reactive.

One of the fundamental osteopathic theories of healing is that structure and function are interrelated, by releasing spinal tension we can have an effect on the internal organ function. Another example of this would be if you slump over a desk and put pressure on your abdomen, the structural shape of your body will affect breathing function and the circulation of blood back to your heart. This inefficient breathing position will further affect your structure. For example, your neck muscles may shorten and tighten as you breathe higher up. Eventually, postural tensions can change the shape of your spine. More pressure may even be placed on the nerves in your neck, further exacerbating the nerve signal for your diaphragm function. How you use your body day to day will add to these tension patterns.

Your body has an amazing ability to compensate and adapt. Pain will tend to occur in the body when it has reached its limit of compensation. This theory means that if you keep your neck moving freely (your structure) the nerve signal to your diaphragm will also be healthy (improved function). Adaptations to tissues can maintain your experience of various conditions even though your body is designed to be self-healing. Your body and breathing will function most efficiently when every part of you is in the best mechanical alignment, there is minimal tension and holding in your body and you breathe gently into your tummy.

Although correct breathing using your diaphragm will reduce the build-up of tension in your neck and shoulders, any old tension may need resolving for you to notice significant improvements. This may take time, depending on the level of tension that has resulted. Massage can help to reduce shoulder and back tension and give you a feeling of relaxation in your body and osteopathy can help to reduce neck, shoulder, ribcage and diaphragm tension. Bowen technique also uses gentle rolling moves which can really help release diaphragm tension. When your body relaxes so does your nervous system and mind; you can be more resourceful with how you respond to the continual demands and pressures of life.

Before you begin the breathing retraining exercises later in this book, it is worth making sure that your body posture and breathing mechanics are functioning well, so you practise effectively. If you are aware of tension around your diaphragm area, there are some simple stretches you can do to aid not only your breathing but your circulation and digestion too.

STEPS TO MASTERY—Week One—Diaphragm Breathing

Continue your ten minutes, twice a day, of breathing into your abdomen. Remember, any time you feel tense breathe down into your tummy, rather than up into your shoulders. You can practise the nose-clearing, neck and diaphragm stretches each day before breathing practice. To stretch and relax the diaphragm, breathe out, pinch your nose and bear down into your abdomen, as though you are trying to pop your ears. Once you feel confident with diaphragm and nose breathing, see if you can add in a twenty-minute walk each day with nose breathing. Remember to stop and regain your nose breathing if you feel breathless. Remember to breathe down into your abdomen keeping your shoulders relaxed.

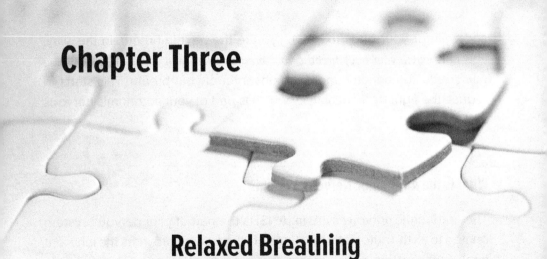

Chapter Three

Relaxed Breathing

Find and remove the cause, then the effect will disappear.

Dr A. T. Still, Founder of Osteopathy[28]

Breathing and the Nervous System

How is your breathing practice going? Some people find that when they focus on their breathing it actually creates more stress and tension and it heightens anxiety. If this is the case, there are a few ways in which you can approach this. You can bring in some creative visualisation, such as taking yourself to your favourite place of relaxation. You could imagine yourself at the beach or in the countryside. We will look at this in greater depth in Part Two. The other way of responding to this is with mini pauses. In Chapter One, the control pause was described as the length of time you could comfortably pause from the end of your out-breath to the next in-breath, as a way of measuring progress. The breath pause will be something to develop and lengthen during your breathing retraining sessions in Part Five. However, mini pauses work well to assist letting go of any tension you create during breathing exercises. For example, after a normal out-breath, pause for a couple of seconds and wait for your body to naturally take the next in-breath. In this way, you can *watch your body breathe your breath rather than you actively breathing your breath*. You become more the observer of your breath. This starts to reduce the fight-or-flight activity which is part of your autonomic nervous system.

What is the Autonomic Nervous System?

The autonomic nervous system (ANS) is the part of your nervous system related to all the automatic functions of your body. It provides the inherent intelligence within your system that coordinates your internal bodily functions, without you even thinking about it. Many of your systems are under both autonomic and conscious control. For example, your body can breathe for you, or you can take over the breathing by thinking about it. Similarly, with a full bladder you can hold on longer if you wish, but ultimately the ANS will decide you can hold no longer and let go. Other organs, such as your heart, can be affected through conscious control; but this takes longer to master and is achieved by focusing more on relaxation than through any physical muscular effort such as moving the ribcage with conscious breathing. Thankfully, you cannot stop your breathing or heart rate voluntarily for any length of time without the ANS kicking in to take over the control.

The ANS picks up information from sensors inside your body which can measure many different variables such as pressure and body chemistry, known as baroreceptors and chemoreceptors. This is why some people may be aware of atmospheric pressure changes affecting how they feel. Some people are sensitive to the chemicals in their environment and those they take in from their diet which affect the nervous system. Your five senses will also feed into how your ANS reacts. This means what you see, feel, smell, taste and hear will affect how your body responds.

Unconscious Breathing and Conscious Retraining

Your breathing is controlled through your nervous system. In your brainstem there are carbon dioxide sensors that cause you to breathe in when CO_2 rises. The brainstem regulates the rate and depth of breathing. The amount of CO_2 in your blood will be determined by the rate at which you breathe and the amount you are exercising. Your brainstem has the majority of breathing control, which with long-term stress may have been set at a faster rate. This hyperventilation causes us to breathe out too much CO_2, causing an imbalance in the system. It is likely that with long-term overbreathing the sensors get used to a lower level of CO_2.

By taking control of your breathing, you start to alter your breathing behaviour, which can be done over a four-week period of time. When you start to retrain your breathing patterns, it is likely to be resetting the sensors in the brainstem to be comfortable with a slightly higher and more normal level of CO_2. When CO_2 is slightly higher, it means that the tissues become better oxygenated because the red blood cells will release oxygen more readily. Whilst doing the breathing exercises it is good to become comfortable with the feeling of a little bit of air hunger. This gradually starts to reduce your drive to breathe, so without even thinking about it your breathing begins to reset to a slower rate.

Sympathetic and Parasympathetic Nervous System

The output from the ANS, the nerves that supply and cause our internal organs to respond to different sensory input, is split into two parts; the sympathetic nervous system (SNS) and the parasympathetic nervous system (PSNS). These nerves can either increase (stimulate) or decrease (inhibit) organ activity, gland secretion and blood vessel dilation and constriction. The SNS responds to *stressful* events and is also associated with the fight-or-flight response which stimulates adrenal gland activity causing the release of adrenaline and cortisol. The PSNS is the *peaceful* part of the autonomic nervous system as it is associated with resting, digesting and elimination. Both the SNS and the PSNS are always working simultaneously, but one side of the nervous system may be more active than the other. When the balance is lost between these two systems, symptoms are usually experienced.

The Sympathetic Nervous System (SNS)

The SNS or fight-or-flight nervous system originates from the thoracic and lumbar spine, forming a chain of nerves deep inside your body core just in front and next to the spinal column close to the rib attachments. Increased breathing can stimulate increased activity in this chain of nerves. The nerves between your shoulder blades, when stimulated, will open the upper airways. The phrenic nerve—which supplies the diaphragm, causing the contraction which expands your lungs—also has sympathetic nerve fibres running through it, which will increase the breathing rate if overstimulated.

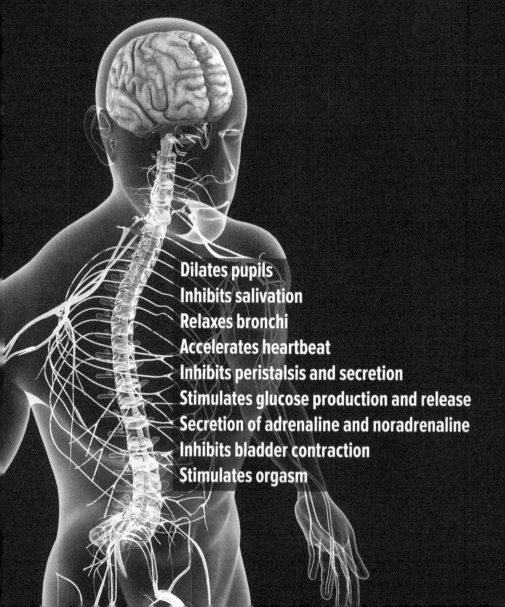

Dilates pupils
Inhibits salivation
Relaxes bronchi
Accelerates heartbeat
Inhibits peristalsis and secretion
Stimulates glucose production and release
Secretion of adrenaline and noradrenaline
Inhibits bladder contraction
Stimulates orgasm

What Happens During a Stress Response?

Increased sympathetic activity elevates heart rate and breathing. Increased breathing rate also increases the SNS stimulation, which in turn stimulates the adrenal glands to produce more adrenaline. This chemically increases heart rate, breathing and increases muscle tension.

The digestive system shuts down as the SNS is stimulated, causing blood vessels to the gut to constrict. This diverts more blood to the muscles, heart and lungs to increase oxygenation, and the liver to break down the sugar stores to increase energy levels. It widens the bronchial passageways, improving oxygenation. Sweating occurs to enable the body to lose the extra heat. In this state, the body is primed for action.

The increased activity within the SNS is also associated with increased tension in the musculoskeletal system, goose bumps, constipation or, if massively overstimulated, can cause a rapid emptying of the bowel and bladder to prevent food and waste from rotting inside us. As the blood vessels in the gut are constricted to divert the blood to the muscles in readiness for fighting or running, it raises the blood pressure in the rest of the system. Over many years of prolonged stress, this can lead to arterial damage along with raised blood sugar which is often converted to fat and deposited in the arteries or tissues. If you are active during this stress response, you burn off the adrenaline and release the nervous tension. It is detrimental to health if you are sedentary in this state.

The interconnection of systems and functions is coordinated by the autonomic nervous system which also controls the different hormones your system releases. We can directly affect the autonomic nervous system through releasing tension in the spinal muscles and muscles around the top and bottom of the spine at the cranium and sacrum. Your breathing rate is also key to working with your body's reactions. By relaxing the central core of your chest at the end of your out-breath you can help reduce the build-up of tension from increased SNS activity.

How do you Experience Stress?

When your stress response is activated, it doesn't necessarily mean you are *aware* of feeling stressed. It can mean that your body's organs are under physiological stress from working long hours, last-minute deadlines, late nights, poor food choices, lack of exercise and unconsciously holding muscle tension in areas of your body. Keeping the body stimulated with caffeine and using alcohol for relaxation requires organs to work harder to eliminate the extra waste. The liver will also have to break down the extra stress hormones whilst the kidneys and bowel eliminate the extra waste. The organ systems can become stressed. Pain will often be experienced with the accumulation of two or three stressors which combine on an emotional, physical or physiological level and give us an early warning that we need to make changes. The experience of pain will also increase the rate of breathing and causes people to hold their in-breath, tensing the body and changing the natural breathing patterns. As pain is heightened by SNS activity, the faster you breathe, the greater the level of pain that can be experienced. Slowing your breathing can reduce your experience of pain.

STEPS TO MASTERY—Week One—Relaxing Your Core

Imagine you can feel into the central core of your body like a column deep inside your chest and abdomen. Have you been holding unconscious tension here? Can feel how to relax and soften this column deep inside your chest and abdomen, especially on your out-breath, letting go of any unnecessary tension. This can help relax your fight-or-flight nervous system. Your whole body relaxes on the out-breath. Imagine your head dropping into your heart to relax your neck and chest.

Have treatment, such as osteopathy, massage, Bowen, acupuncture to reduce remaining tension in the whole of your body and choose a class from gentle yoga, Pilates, Tai Chi, Feldenkrais or Alexander Technique to aid the correct movement of your spine and ribcage. Make sure your ribcage is directly above your pelvis when you breathe. When sitting at a desk, be aware of where your head is positioned. If your head moves forwards, your upper back muscles will tighten to hold your head up.

The Relaxation Response and the Parasympathetic Nervous System

The parasympathetic nervous system arises from the top and bottom of the spine, which is what we try to influence with cranio-sacral osteopathy, which aids the relaxation of your nervous system by supporting the PSNS activity. The PSNS is made up of the two cranial nerves known as the *vagus nerves*, and the *pelvic nerves,* which exit around the sacrum at the base of the spine.

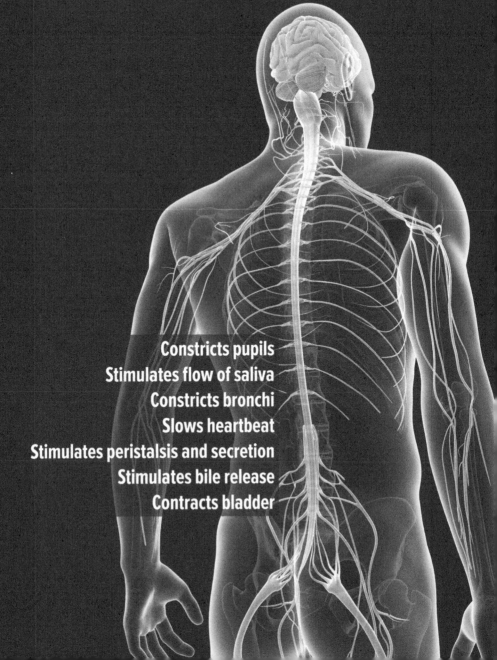

Constricts pupils
Stimulates flow of saliva
Constricts bronchi
Slows heartbeat
Stimulates peristalsis and secretion
Stimulates bile release
Contracts bladder

The vagus nerves, which exit at the base of your skull, outside of the spinal column, feed sensory information back to the brainstem and can also actively stimulate or inhibit the organ smooth muscle or motor activity in the body. The vagus nerves supply the heart, lungs, stomach and most of the intestines. Vagal activity slows down the breathing and heart rate and encourages digestion and elimination of waste. Branches of these two nerves stimulate the stomach to produce acid and the wave-like motion of peristalsis to move food through the digestive system.

The PSNS nerves that arise from the pelvis are also associated with the functioning of your reproductive organs and the muscles in the wall of your bowel at the end of the large intestine. Both the cranial and pelvic nerves are associated with the production of mucus, tears and saliva. If you cry, you have switched out of fight-or-flight dominance and into vagal dominance. During an asthma attack, it is likely that the sympathetic dominance has been lost and the increased vagal activity—which increases mucus production and constricts the smooth muscle of the bronchi—is responsible.[29] Usually, a deep breath will open up the airways, but with asthma there is a failure of deep inspiration to open the airways,[30] possibly because the vagus is further stimulated by the stretch in the lung tissues. This is why fighting the constriction with deeper breathing doesn't work to relieve an attack. See if you can consciously breathe small-volume, quiet breaths into your abdomen rather than large-volume, deep breaths. This should help to reduce the overactivity of the vagal tone.

Vagal tone is still important in the general health of the body, as it also helps to reduce chronic inflammation in the rest of the body.[31, 32] Inducing the relaxation response in your body is also mediated by the vagal tone or activity. Making sure there is just enough vagal tone is key. Keeping your stress levels to a minimum with slow, relaxed breathing can help prevent a crisis situation.

When you are in good health both parts of the ANS work in harmony with one another. There is a natural equilibrium between the coordinated functioning of the SNS and PSNS to maintain homeostasis in the body. At some stages there will be an increase in the SNS activity and at other times, an increase in PSNS activity. If one side of the ANS becomes dominant through overactivity for a prolonged period of time and then becomes exhausted, dis-ease can occur. The body is still working as a whole, but it is responding in the best way it can under the circumstances.

There is a way of measuring the balance of activity between the PSNS and SNS through heart rate variability (HRV) biofeedback studies. As you breathe in the heart speeds up, and as you breathe out the heart slows down. This natural phenomenon is known as *respiratory sinus arrhythmia*. You might be able to experience this by noticing the speed of your wrist pulse as you breathe in and out. HRV measurements typically show decreased SNS activity and increased PSNS activity in people with asthma, especially when it is uncontrolled.[33] Respiratory sinus arrhythmia is very noticeable in young people and athletes but less so as we age. HRV measures this speeding up and slowing down of the heart rate with breathing and the better the HRV reading, the better the balance of the SNS and PSNS. By using the diaphragm to breathe with minimal chest expansion, it possibly acts to stimulate the sympathetic fibres in the phrenic and calm the vagus by not overexpanding the lungs.

There is a third control of the lungs via part of your nervous system that doesn't respond to either the SNS or PSNS activity—the NANC nervous system. These receptors respond to nitric oxide gas (NO),[34] which is produced when you nose breathe. As the sympathetic nerves only control the opening of the upper airways, the deeper lung tissue is only dilated by nitric oxide through this third system, which is why nose breathing is so important to keep your airways open. The spray used in angina creates NO in the body and helps to dilate the arteries in the heart. It is also what is released by drugs used commonly for erectile dysfunction. Although we can't say that nose breathing will cure these issues, it can certainly help maintain healthy breathing which keeps the body functioning optimally.

You can encourage a reduction in the overstimulation of the vagus by releasing tension around the base of the skull and neck to normalise function. If you focus your attention on your sitting bones or feet and think about relaxing into this area, it can help to ground your body and calm you and reduce stress and neck tension. Walking in the dew is another grounding activity which is very calming for your body. If tension has been long-standing and has built up significantly, you may need a helping hand to release the tension through physical treatment. Once the background level of tension has been released, you will be able to notice the relaxation response more easily. We are aiming for relaxation, not exhaustion—which is what happens during an asthma attack.

Relaxing in the Breath Pause

The breath pause, or breath hold time, has been shown to be lower in people who chest breathe and have lower spirometry readings,[35] which measures the amount and speed of your exhale. The length of breath hold is also a good indicator of how much shortness of breath or air hunger is being experienced.[36] Although the breath pause (or control pause) is used as a measure of progress, by lengthening the time you can pause it helps to relax the nervous system in relation to the feeling of air hunger and reset your breathing. With practice, it is possible to experience the chest tension relaxing as you do this. The more you can relax and soften into the pause the better the response will be. Pausing at the end of your out-breath in a relaxed way allows your whole system to rest. When you give yourself time to rest, the exhausted parts of your system have time to recover. Balance can once again be restored.

In people with chronic fatigue, paced breathing at a slower rate has been shown to reduce vagal tone[37], which gives an explanation as to why it is helpful in an asthmatic situation. It has also been shown that poor HRV readings are associated with chest breathing rather than diaphragm breathing at rest.[38] Whether there is raised sympathetic or vagal tone, relaxed breathing will hopefully have the effect of simply normalising both sides of the ANS as your body always tries to take the most intelligent response it can, given your current situation. If you change any aspect of your life, it will have an effect on the whole. How conscious you are of the choices you make, will inform the wellness you express and experience. Wherever you find yourself you can always increase the depth of your experience of health and wholeness.

STEPS TO MASTERY—Week One—Quiet Breathing

Making your breathing as quiet as possible enables your body to start relaxing. If you place your finger under your nostrils, the airflow shouldn't be that noticeable. If you can feel a strong stream of air against your finger, you are breathing too much. Whilst retraining your breathing it is necessary to start to become comfortable with the feeling of a little bit of air hunger. The more comfortable and relaxed you can be with this feeling the greater the progress you will make. Notice where in your body you need to soften, to achieve this relaxation.

Tension in your body will relate to challenges within your ANS. This week notice how much tension you use during simple daily tasks such as brushing your teeth, holding the steering wheel, or even washing the dishes. Become aware of how you hold tension in your body. Scan your body and notice any other areas of holding. When you notice an area of tension, you can let the area relax on the out-breath.

Imagine a balloon attached to the top of your head to enable it to feel like it can float on the top of your spine. This will relieve pressure on both the vagus and your sympathetic nerves. Bring your attention to the base of your spine and support your lower back, to help relax your neck.

PART TWO—
THE EMOTIONS

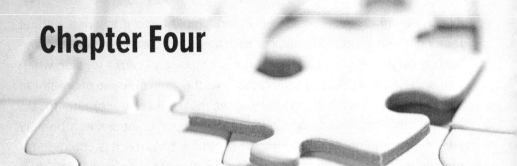

Chapter Four

Your Body and Emotions

New beginnings are often disguised as painful endings.

Lao Tzu

Emotion and the Breath

You cannot separate your body from your emotions, as your body is where you register your emotions. You may have noticed that when emotions arise breathing becomes more rapid or you may stop breathing altogether. If you try to resist being emotional, by holding your breath, it is likely you will build up tension in your body, especially your diaphragm, ribcage and shoulders. Although feelings and emotions may seem very intangible, you can get a sense of where you feel them by scanning your body as you experience them. For example, when you feel sadness, it is likely that you feel it in the chest or throat. It is more often the case that when we feel a strong emotion and try to resist what we are feeling, we will have a stronger sense of where we feel it in the body. You may find yourself breathing higher and higher in your chest to avoid feeling emotional discomfort arising from your solar plexus, just below your diaphragm.

If you feel an emotion, welcome it and simply allow it to arise without feeding it with a story. The lack of resistance will mean it is free to come and go very easily. Emotions only remain stuck and cause tension when you resist them and keep feeding them. As the main purpose of breathing training to overcome asthma is finding ways to reduce your breathing rate and breathe into your tummy, working with your emotions in a healthy way is fundamental to recovering your natural balance. It is common for many people to suppress emotions to the point of overwhelm, and then it is like having an overflowing bucket, which simply needs emptying for us to feel well again.

There are four emotional locks that you may be using to prevent yourself from feeling your emotions, but in reality, any emotion you resist will have tension associated with it in any area of your body, including the organs, muscles or joints. Where you tense in relation to an emotion will be related to where the feeling registers in your body and will likely predispose you to have symptoms there, as blood flow and oxygenation will be reduced.

The Four Emotional Locks

The four emotional locks correspond with the four diaphragms. The word diaphragm originates from the Greek *dia* meaning *apart* or *through* and *phragma* meaning *fence*. You only have one true breathing diaphragm, but the other three diaphragms are simply muscles which horizontally divide sections of the body. The breathing diaphragm separates the thoracic and abdominal cavity. We also have a pelvic diaphragm or the pelvic floor which stops our organs descending through the pelvic outlet. At the top of the ribcage, we have the thoracic inlet which has muscles covering the top of the thorax at the base of the neck. We also have membranes in the base of our skull which divide sections of our brain and prevent it dropping through the opening in the base of the cranium.

An example of using an emotional lock is buttock clenching if you are feeling stressed, which locks away fear and vulnerability. This can tighten the hips and cause problems emptying the bladder or bowel. Next time you are driving fast down the motorway or washing the dishes whilst thinking of the hundred and one things you feel you also need to do, just check to see if you are clenching your buttocks and let them go. Bringing your awareness to the present moment will also help reduce the strain on your system.

If you are dealing with emotional stress, you may tighten your breathing diaphragm to resist feeling what you are feeling in the solar plexus. The solar plexus is known as the seat of emotions. It is where you may have felt *butterflies* in your stomach if you are nervous, along with other emotions such as anger and frustration. If you are *shouldering* responsibility and feel burdened, you might tighten the thoracic inlet and shoulder girdle. Fear of not being loved, along with grief, loss and aloneness will all register in the chest area. Resisting feeling these emotions as we pull ourselves together to carry on will create chest and shoulder tension. If you are worrying or overthinking, you are likely to tighten the membranes in the cranium.

The key to unlocking these areas is to imagine breathing into each part of your body and softening it as you relax on the out-breath. All the muscles in the body relax as you breathe out, allowing the emotions to flow through unimpeded. If you use the breath pause at the end of the out-breath, you can imagine surrendering into what you are feeling. Surrender doesn't mean giving up; it simply means not wanting it to be any different from how it is happening.

If you find yourself in a stressful situation, for example when you next sit in the dentist's chair, scan your body and see if you are holding tension anywhere. You may well have a signature holding pattern that repeats during stressful events. Learning to catch this and allowing yourself to relax, will make a big difference in enabling your nervous system and breathing to remain calm. Grounding yourself is one of the most powerful things you can do to relax. Sink right down into your bottom and allow your head and neck to rest, and your tummy and shoulders to soften.

Your Emotions and Your Health

There is nothing wrong with feeling emotions. They can be indicators of your desire for something different and may have their roots in early childhood or past experience. Your emotions are a good indicator of how well your thoughts or beliefs and experience are aligned. You may be able to identify limiting beliefs through the emotions you are experiencing. In order to resolve the emotional tension, you need to close the gap between where you are and where you would like to be. If you can identify the belief or story that is feeding the emotion, you can imagine that you are letting this old idea go on the out-breath, surrendering in the pause and then breathe in a new more empowering belief in its place. Have compassion for what you are feeling; it is not wrong, it can be an act of letting go of what is past so that something better can arise in its place. Have compassion for yourself, even in your darkest moments. The only person you can truly love unconditionally is you.

If what you are feeling has been brought to the surface through your interaction with someone else, know that whatever you feel about them, your body is feeling about you, which may give you an indication of your limiting beliefs. For example, if you are feeling abandoned, how have you abandoned yourself? Having gratitude for them highlighting this situation so that you can free yourself from your past limitations enables you to move into a future that has greater freedom. They are not mirroring how you treat others, they are mirroring how you treat yourself. Love will bring to the surface everything unlike itself to be healed.

Freezing and Thawing

You are probably familiar with the fight-or-flight response to stress. However, there is a third response known as the freeze response. This is what happens when our body stays tense and restricted and won't easily release following prolonged stress or a sudden shock. It's a bit like the rabbit in the headlights.

In *Waking the Tiger: Healing Trauma*, Peter Levine gives a great analogy of how animals release shock so that they don't become traumatised. He describes a cheetah chasing an antelope. As the chase is going on around seventy miles an hour, just as the cheetah is about to pounce, the antelope drops to the ground in the freezing response. This has two benefits. It prevents the antelope from feeling pain at the point of death. If the cheetah thinks he has killed the antelope and hasn't, it gives it a chance to escape at a later point in time.

Internally it is a bit like having the accelerator on at seventy miles per hour whilst also having the break on at the same time. There is a huge amount of nervous energy that will be whirling around in the solar plexus region, not being discharged. If the cheetah takes his catch back to his lair and then walks off, it gives the antelope a chance to escape. It can then go through a reorientation process, where it shakes and shivers and discharges all the nervous energy and runs away untraumatised.

Unfortunately, when humans experience a traumatic event we often hold it together and maintain the internal tension which can create a freezing response. It is most important that if you have experienced a shock that you allow yourself time to release it. Sometimes old shock can surface at the time we are experiencing a stressful event in the present. In this way the current event can be used to free up the old tension that has been holding us captive so that we can move forwards in freedom. Shock or trauma can be held in our body for decades. Tears and laughter both create involuntary shaking, shivering responses, which is our body's natural way of releasing shock. Even standing and shaking your body, keeping your feet on the ground is a good way to release tension as you breathe out. If you experience an event with similar emotional content to something from your past, it gives you an opportunity to respond differently. Try physically shaking the issue out. Doing this to music can make it more fun.

Laughter can trigger asthmatic breathing, so it is important to have a prolonged exhale and then as you breathe in, make sure it is a slow belly breath rather than high up in the chest and neck. Avoid tensing the front of your neck as you breathe in. When we have an emotional shock, we have faster breathing and faster heart rate. When we are having fun, we also have faster breathing and heart rate. Our brain can become confused between the two and so can constrict in a protective freezing response in relation to the happy event. Allow yourself to experience joy and excitement by relaxing and softening your body and staying grounded. You can imagine your heart space opening and expanding in the pause and allowing the feeling of joy and love to spread through you rather than resisting it.

Often when we start to relax more, old emotions can surface. We don't need to sift through them too much, just be grateful that the old tension is releasing. I found that if I cried whilst I was wheezing it would relieve the asthmatic symptoms. This isn't a long-term solution, but it does indicate that a build-up of emotional tension in the body is probably responsible, especially if we have ignored how we have been feeling for a while, to the point of overwhelm. As crying is a parasympathetic response, similar to bronchial constriction, releasing the tears may release some of the vagal overactivity. The involuntary shaking action going through the chest and shoulders whilst crying may well be thawing out some of the unconscious holding. As asthma is often seen as a condition of breathing in too much and not breathing out, the act of crying is one of letting go with the out-breath with a prolonged pause that switches us out of hyperventilation. You don't need to feed the tears, but know that it is ok to let go.

Sometimes if we have held on to emotional tension for too long, it can make us ill. Stress depletes our immune system. How you handle this healing crisis is going to make a difference as to how you heal and recover. Suppression often causes a more chronic health situation to develop. You will learn how to go through a healing crisis naturally in Part Three.

Grief and the Lungs

The 1918-1920 flu pandemic, at the end of the First World War, is a good example of how illness and stress are linked. Traditional Chinese medicine associates the lungs with grief, and at a time when grief would have been a worldwide experience, people's immune system would have been under the greatest strain. One third of the world's population, around 500 million people were affected, and around 20-50 million people died; more than in the war itself. Around this time there were osteopathic hospitals in America that treated patients with flu and had significantly lower mortality than the medical hospitals. The overall mortality rate in the hospitals was around 30% whereas the mortality rate in the osteopathic hospitals was around 0.25% with just under 2,500 osteopaths treating over 110,000 patients successfully, which in many cases presented as pneumonia. [39, 40] The medical hospitals were using cough syrup and aspirin which lowered temperature. The body creates a high temperature as a necessary part of fighting the infection. The osteopathic hospitals didn't use aspirin but applied osteopathic treatment to improve drainage and circulation and improve the tissue oxygenation, using chest pumping, rib stretching and pumping of the lymphatic system to aid recovery.

Managing the Emotional Crisis

When we are ill, it is often the case that all the emotions that we have suppressed during everyday life have the opportunity to surface. It is usually once we are off the battlefield that we feel our symptoms more, as this is when our natural anti-inflammatories drop, and the body starts to eliminate the waste that was kept in storage during the crisis period, creating a fertile breeding ground for virus and bacteria to grow. Once this waste has been eliminated, there is often a resetting of the system which can enable a return to better health. You might find your control pause increases, or it is easier to breathe through your nose or your lungs feel clearer, once the old waste has been thoroughly eliminated. Using your slow breathing and avoiding coughing too much can help you get through your crisis. Many people I have worked with that have used the breathing techniques have found that they don't go through their usual autumn cold or chest infections as they usually do. They produce less mucus because they are not hyperventilating any more.

Positive Affirmations

At the start of any journey, it is a good idea to set an intention for where you would like to go. Otherwise, we could go round in circles. Whilst focusing on your emotions it is a good time to set a positive intention or affirmation as to what you would like to achieve. Affirmations work best when you already have the feeling of having what you intend, not when you see it at some distant point in the future. If you catch yourself worrying about your health or something in your life, as soon as you catch yourself, affirm that all will be well, or take the necessary action to move in that direction.

In order for healing to happen, you need to regain trust in your body again. If there has been a health problem, we can often feel let down by our body. Learning to listen to your body's needs so that you can trust yourself once more is top priority. Having enough self-worth to take good care of yourself is essential for recovery. Going through life fearing things will only maintain the problem. Affirming something positive will set a course of action. Similar to reprogramming a computer, affirmations can help to change your internal programming that may be causing or maintaining a malfunction and help restore normal functioning once more.

If trusting your breathing is too big a leap at the moment, you can do it in simple stages. Having experienced my worst health just after completing my osteopathy degree, having indulged in too many biscuits, cheese, chocolate, stressful deadlines, late nights and emotional rollercoasters for too many years, I injured my knee. Although it was a mechanical injury, there had been a lot of emotional stress in my life at the time it happened and whenever I thought of the stress I could feel the pain in my knee being triggered. This taught me a lot about healing and recovery and how emotions can be linked with our physical body. Have you noticed any emotional states being linked to the symptoms you experience?

I noticed that I would get frustrated with the inability to be able to do the physical activities that I wanted to do. This was compounded by imagining a future of inactivity and pain. It was after an acupuncture treatment with one of my colleagues that I suddenly realised what I was doing to prevent the healing. From a new perspective I recognised that the future hadn't happened yet; it was unwritten and it could be what I made it.

If I started picturing a future where my knee recovered then I was more likely to heal, than remaining in my doom and gloom. Recognising that our knees need to flex in order for us to move forwards, I saw this as a symbolic injury around my fear of moving forwards in my life. I took myself on a walking holiday in Scotland on my own. Any time I sensed the fear of pain starting to creep in, I immediately stated, *"My knees are strong and flexible and I move freely forwards."* Having regained my confidence on a moderate walk, I decided to walk twenty miles and also ran up and down Ben Nevis using walking poles in complete comfort. I knew my knee was better and I trusted it once more.

You can approach your respiratory health in the same way. Start to picture a future where your breathing is improving, and any time fear of your breathing issue arises, know you can easily release your emotional tension in the pause at the end of the out-breath. You may even begin to feel worthy of asking for your needs to be met rather than being responsible for everyone else. Caring about yourself enough to practise the exercises and make your health top priority is essential.

To create a positive affirmation, create a statement that is positively phrased in the present tense and feel what it feels like to already have achieved this new reality.

Your subconscious doesn't hear negatives. If someone tells you *not* to think of pink elephants, you don't start thinking of blue ones—well you are now! But you see what I mean. Saying, "My breathing is *not* wheezy," is not a positive affirmation, as the statement is about the wheeze, not about the relief or the improvement. Start imagining a reality where you too can breathe with ease and then take the necessary action to make this a reality.

The affirmation becomes a statement of intent, and it is important that we believe in what we are saying and have a positive feeling behind the intention. If you feel what you are saying doesn't have a positive emotion behind it or feels like a lie, then take a small step like, "Every day my breathing is improving." You can also thank your body for the healing that is happening and for giving yourself time to do your breathing practice. Have a clear idea of what you would like the positive outcome to be and how that would make you feel. The intention that I set many years ago was, "I Breathe with Ease." I had no idea that it would involve writing a book. Be careful what you wish for!

Stating your intention to a friend or writing it down will add power to your affirmation as it has been witnessed. It could also be something like, *"When I see a cat or dog I relax my breathing and soften my chest."* Catching thoughts just before they take hold and then changing them enables you to transform your reality, similar to changing your thoughts from a blue elephant back to a pink elephant, or whatever you choose.

Secondary Gains

Secondary gains are the benefits we derive from being unwell. Maybe we gain more attention when we are unwell, than when we are healthy, maybe we use our health as an excuse for whether we attend a social function. Becoming ill on the day of a big event or something we don't want to do is a way of self-sabotaging. It is better to say *no* in the first place or work out what your fear is and release this so that you can fully commit to your word to enjoy and maintain high-level health.

Fear

The emotional locks or tension we experience during stress are due to fear or resisting fear. There can be many different aspects to fear; fear of the unknown, fear of failure, fear of exposure, fear of getting hurt, fear of not being loved and even fear of fear itself, which compounds the experience! Fear in itself won't kill you, it is how we react to the fear that causes us problems. If you have ever experienced an asthma attack or panic attack, the struggle to catch your breath can be quite frightening. One fear that often arises for people during this time is the fear of death and dying.

The Breakthrough

As allergic asthma is something that you can avoid by not exposing yourself to allergens, I did a pretty good job of keeping myself out of contact, which was necessary for me to remain well. During my early twenties, I saw a therapist, called Barry Male, who did guided meditations and helped me learn how to breathe properly into my abdomen. Barry had cats, which initially I saw as a distinct disadvantage, and often led me to wheeze during our sessions.

One day I was lying on the couch, wheezing away with an allergic asthmatic response, struggling to catch my breath. As he guided me into the meditation that day, in my mind's eye I unexpectedly felt transported back to medieval times, being walked along a path to a river. I felt a certain foreboding as I was walked over to where the ducking stool was placed by the river. As I was sat on the stool, I felt as though I was being ducked under water. With my eyes closed and chest tighter than ever, I felt like I was drowning as I went under the water. I have never had a drowning experience in this lifetime, but it felt so incredibly real. Barry guided me by suggesting that I just surrendered to the water.

The feeling of being short of breath brings us face to face with the fear of our mortality, and many anxiety states bring us to this point. As I struggled and fought against the feeling of tension in my chest trying to inflate my lungs against massive resistance, Barry instructed me to just let go. I felt something inside me soften, as though I had surrendered to the drowning feeling. It felt like surrendering to death.

I had passed into a different time and space and was held in the watery embrace of eternity. I had become one with the water around me. The experience of bliss following the struggle was sublime. I no longer feared my mortality; there was no fear in this space. My whole body relaxed into the water, I didn't have to breathe my breath any more, my breath felt like it would go on forever.

As the tension had spontaneously dissolved, my breath started effortlessly breathing itself. It felt like my breath or my spirit was timeless, effortless, free, connected with the flowing water all around me. The wheeze had completely dissolved the instant I surrendered. I was filled with peace deeper than I had ever experienced before.

Whether my experience was a past life or a genetic memory or simply a construct that my mind created to help heal itself, it doesn't really matter. For me what mattered was the breakthrough. I had switched from full-blown wheeze to normal breathing in a matter of seconds and was still in the presence of animals.

It took me seven more years before I was able to consciously reproduce the same effect that I had spontaneously experienced during my healing session that day as I surrendered and let go. By the time I learnt how to release my wheeze consciously, I had also discovered the necessary tools to enable my healing and to facilitate other people's healing process too, which I felt inspired to share with you.

Meditation is a little like taking a jar of sandy water and letting it settle so that you have clear water separate from the sand. When we face an emotion during meditation and we surrender to what we are experiencing, it can enable you to sieve the sand from the water and find the gold in the sand, as well as maintaining clearer water, even when shaken. Clearing old issues allows you to make present-day changes and you will find yourself responding differently to similar situations.

Love

It might be an obvious statement, but the antidote to fear is love. Love is an expansive feeling and something you can become open to experiencing in your breath pauses. Whilst you pause, you can bring your attention to your heart space and imagine any tension expanding outwards. One of the most amazing discoveries is that the electromagnetic field around the heart is 100 to 1,000 times stronger than the field around the brain.[41] You don't have to work out how to be well, it is a natural state of being that is often buried underneath all the surface stuff we have accumulated through our lives. Give greater importance to your heartfelt feelings than your thoughts. In the softening of your heart centre and expanding your awareness in the pause you can access love inside of you, for you, and know that you are love. The love that is your true essence can never be destroyed and is the truth of who you really are.

STEPS TO MASTERY—Week Two—Affirmations and Breathing into What you Feel

Formulate a personal affirmation that enables you to start feeling you can already breathe with ease. You can apply this to any area of your life, not just your breathing. Connect with your heart in the pause, allowing a warm feeling to spread through your chest. Then, as you do your daily breathing practice, if any old memories present themselves, imagine you can stand right behind the *you* in that memory and give yourself in that memory the love and support that you may not have been able to access at the time. If wheezing shows up, give compassion even to the vulnerable parts of you. Scan your body from head to toe and release any areas of unconscious holding. If an area feels resistant to change, return to it later.

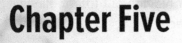

Chapter Five

Overcoming Anger—

Finding a Route Through the Storm

Anyone can become angry—that is easy,

but to be angry with the right person and to the right degree

and at the right time and for the right purpose and in the right

way—that is not within everybody's power and is not easy.

Aristotle

Your Emotional Fight-or-Flight

In our modern society, we don't appear to deal with our anger much better than our ancestors did in the time of Aristotle. With asthma and many other inflammatory health conditions, many emotions are internalised. Breathing can become more restricted when internal emotions are different from what is presented externally. There is an enormous tension created when your outside appearance is not congruent with how you really feel inside. By putting on a front or hiding your true feelings, you often negate your darker or shadow aspects.

Anything that you sit on will inevitably drain your energy and create extra stress for your system. Long-term suppression of anger can cause depression and symptoms in the body.[42,43] This takes energy that can be better used for daily living. Living a more authentic life requires noticing how you feel. Shining a light on your darker aspects brings them out of the shadows and into the light so you can become conscious of how you really feel. You don't have to act out what you feel, simply acknowledging it and being willing to either let the feeling go or breathe through what you are feeling is enough to give you greater freedom from these emotional tensions. Breathing through your feelings and having them witnessed is helpful to release tensions associated with emotional stress.

All of your emotions will change how you breathe. We often talk casually of the fight-or-flight response, but what does that really have to do with your emotional state? The fight response will tend to produce anger, frustration and defensiveness, the flight response is more associated with fear, anxiety and avoidance. Anger can be more enabling and help us approach and overcome adversity, but only if short-lived. A recent study looking at the blood chemistry associated with both anger and anxiety states showed that it was anxiety that was more prone to increase inflammatory markers in the bloodstream.[44]

Anger tends to be a more expansive energy if it's not suppressed. Fear tends to be more constrictive. If we don't face what we are feeling, the fear of our emotions creates a further layer of anxiety, so the tension builds. What you feel on the surface isn't necessarily what you feel deep down. For example, if a car cut someone up on the road whilst driving their car, most people would react with anger, but the underlying emotion would be a fear for their life; an anxiety response, masked by anger.

Breathing patterns also change with different emotions. If you feel afraid, you are more likely to breathe more rapidly. When you feel joy and freedom, there is an ease and flow to your breathing. With deep peace your breath can feel expanded and open as though it just breathes itself. In this state, you experience your authentic self. It may help to recognise that many other emotions we experience are based on a lie or mistaken belief. Your more challenging, uncomfortable emotions can stand in the way of experiencing the ease in your mind and body which is reflected in your breathing. If you can allow yourself to experience life fully without contracting or tensing your body in an attempt to self-protect, you will breathe through your emotions more effortlessly than if you were resisting what you are feeling. This takes practice.

Frustration

Frustration is an emotion often experienced when you feel stuck or unable to move forwards in your life or achieve the health you would like. The emotional tension that this frustration creates adds to the overall physical tension and holding in the body. Add also the unresolved emotional tension that contributed to the condition in the first place with the fear of not recovering and we create a maintaining factor.

There is a world of difference between *feeling* frustrated and *acknowledging* that you are feeling frustrated. When you acknowledge how you are feeling, you have the power of choice. Simply accepting where you are right now, removes the struggle with yourself. It doesn't mean this is how it will always be, it is just where you are right now.

Avoidance Strategies

Often strong or uncomfortable emotions are avoided because they feel unpleasant. You cannot stop yourself from feeling unpleasant emotions, although I tried for many years by living more in my head. When you live in judgement, you disconnect from how you feel in your body. It works to a point as an avoidance strategy but, sooner or later, all the feelings catch up with us and that's often when we experience overwhelm or exhaustion. People run all kinds of behaviours to avoid feeling what they feel. For example, watching television, distracting yourself with mindless internet surfing, stuffing emotions down with food, blaming others or artificially stimulating yourself with chocolate, caffeine and refined sugar, using alcohol to relax, and working too much. The wheeze at the end of the day can occur simply because we have overworked. Seeing these behaviours and judging them in others is often more comfortable than confronting what you feel within yourself.

Bottled up anger can often become held in the abdomen by tensing the diaphragm, which can also cause the neck to tighten in response as we brace ourselves and breathe more in our upper chest. Persistent irritating coughs can be a way that we bark at the world when something is not fully expressed. If you have a belly full of anger, deep breathing is often challenging. So why would you want to face emotions such as anger, jealousy or loneliness? The opposite of these emotions is what most people really want to experience; the peace, joy and oneness that reside in your core self.

Over a prolonged period of time, it may contribute to many different health conditions, including inflammation, arthritic conditions, high blood pressure, tension headaches, blood sugar fluctuations, even weight gain, as comfort eating can happen as a way of numbing our angry belly. If we feel ashamed of our emotions and behaviours, this shame will also keep us trapped and prevent us from experiencing our true essence. It is ok to feel how you feel.

Finding Freedom Through Emotions

It is not possible to heal and become whole if you are dissociated from parts of yourself. Avoiding strong emotions simply maintains stress and tension within your system. There is no freedom in being constantly on the run. Similarly, being perpetually angry and defensive is draining; it keeps love and joy at bay. Rather than suppressing what you feel, releasing emotions in a healthy way can bring you back to discovering your underlying essence. In this place you are more resourced to recognise belief systems that are a lie, such as I am unworthy, not good enough, unlovable, a failure and so on. When you are connected to your truth, you will recognise you are worthy, you are lovable, there is no failure, you can grow from your experiences and you *are* enough. By clearing the stored emotions, there is more space inside for the joy and peace to express itself through you.

Most times when we resist emotions or even pain in the body we try to minimise them. This often creates more tension and holding and prevents the body from integrating what we are feeling. If good blood flow and oxygenation are required to heal, by creating more tension through resistance, we simply prevent our own healing. This applies as much to resisting an illness as an emotion. Acceptance is a good starting point. By accepting and welcoming what you are feeling and expanding the feeling outwards, you start to dissolve the intensity of it and release the tension around it so that your body can heal and integrate that part. The relief you can feel by being willing to face your emotions and breathe through them enables you to access the peace, happiness and love that is your true essence.

When you recognise an emotion that is surfacing, you can ask yourself, "What would I have to believe in order to feel this way?" What is the unhealthy "I am ..." statement or story that is feeding the emotion? Whatever you state after "I am..." is the most powerfully creative statement you can make and creates a belief. A belief is only a thought you have repeated often to yourself. As soon as you become aware of it, it no longer has such power over you to create your reality. Once you are in a more positive emotional state, you can choose to reach for a new belief or understanding about who you are.

When a thought is associated with an emotion, it is more powerful, just as in the affirmations. You don't have to keep checking your thoughts all the time as your emotions are powerful indicators of what you are feeling and believing. By releasing uncomfortable emotions and coming to rest in a more heart centred, loving space you are also releasing limiting beliefs. Once you have released the stored emotions through your breath, without acting from them, you will be more able to recognise the lie you have been telling yourself. Being able to feel these emotions and welcoming them without acting from them is the aim. Whilst you are breathing through an emotion, accepting it means not trying to change it or fix it whilst you are breathing through it. Just have the intention of allowing it to expand outwards. Eventually, it will release.

The Unconscious Programming

Often women are brought up to be *good girls*. When they feel anger, it is deemed unacceptable. When women are not fully empowered, anger often gets switched into tears and confused with sadness. Some believe that wheezing is a sign of suppressed tears. On the other hand, many men are taught not to feel their emotions, especially sadness. The idea that *big boys don't cry* means they have to hold it all in. Anger can create a boundary in order to resist feeling more vulnerable emotions. When these emotions surface repeatedly, it may be driven by a subconscious belief of not being good enough. Being willing to feel your vulnerability in relation to this will enable you to experience unconditional love for you, just as you are. When you are willing to feel your vulnerability, whilst staying grounded, you can be more open to experience love and connect with your essence, which is where you will experience your greatest joy and freedom.

Finding the love on the inside is the most important step you can take. Love, in this definition, is like the energy that holds all of life, not the mushy romantic stuff, although that is an aspect of it. Our loved ones enable us to open our hearts more fully. You are not your emotions, they are something that passes through you. If the truth of who you are in your essence is love and freedom, you are the sky and your emotions are like clouds. The sun is always shining on the other side of the clouds. We can make the mistake of identifying ourselves with the clouds, but, in reality, you are the sky. Either way, you simply have to wait for the clouds to disperse or go through them to reconnect with the sunshine and open sky.

If you have felt under the weather and feelings of hopelessness or helplessness surface during bouts of difficulty breathing, the emotion of anger is a step in a positive direction. It is not to suggest that you stay angry or wallow in the emotion, more that you simply touch the emotion and breathe through it and connect with the power behind this as you surf the wave. Getting tumbled in the wave can happen, but in time you can learn to surf the wave and experience your inner joy. An emotion can pass by in only a couple of minutes if you let go of the story and are willing to simply feel and experience what you are feeling.

Accessing Your Life Force

There is a significant difference between a surface feeling of calm and true peace. Peace has a depth that runs through the whole of you. The problem with being calm is it is often only surface deep. There can be a whole well of unexpressed and suppressed feelings as we try to hold it all together through daily life, especially if you have avoided confronting problem situations. Stepping into your authentic power, rather than simply allowing the angst to fester inside, is essential.

Present-day situations which trigger old stored emotions can be a gift, although it might not feel like that when it happens. These experiences give you a chance to be able to access any unresolved emotional pain and approach it from a new perspective. It is important to bring your awareness into your body so you can begin to notice where you feel your emotions. It is a good practice to scan your body to identify exactly where you feel what you feel. Being curious about this process will prevent you getting sucked into a potential quagmire of emotion. As you welcome what you feel without identifying yourself as the emotion, the emotion can pass quite quickly. It is only when we become invested in feeling the way we do that it sticks. Every negative emotion is your potential power that has been blocked. The emotion can be an opening for you to reconnect with your inner power.

When we experience our inner power, if we are not comfortable feeling it, we will run avoidance behaviour. For example, if you have witnessed people abuse their power and found it uncomfortable, then it is likely that you won't want to tap into your own personal power. However, power doesn't have to be used abusively. If it is used with an open heart, it can be a powerful force for change. Anger is often thought of as a negative emotion. However, before emotion is linked with behaviour, it is simply a powerful potential energy; one which can create change and enable us to move into a new reality. For example, you might have seen the frustration that toddlers experience when they attempt to walk or crawl for the first time. It takes enormous energy and determination. Anger is not necessarily power, but behind anger there is a powerful life force. If we resist anger, it can block us from accessing our life force. Sometimes emotions can feel like clouds and other times they feel like tidal waves.

If the emotion is a wave, then your aim is to connect with the power of the ocean behind the wave.

The Gift in the Present

If you feel someone or something has triggered an angry response in you, it may well be a gift. If angry people show up in your life, it is likely that there is some inner anger festering inside, or you are set in a programme that requires someone to wake you up to get fired up about a situation. Present-day situations may have a similar resonance to a past emotional experience that hasn't been fully resolved. These triggers help you to get access to suppressed or subconscious emotions so that you can release them and discover a new truth. Whatever triggers you to experience an emotional reaction can also give you access to your beliefs and programmes without having to dig. Although they can be painful, once you have released this stored hurt or pain through the breath work, and resolved the underlying mistaken belief you don't need to face it again. If the same emotions and situation keep presenting themselves, there may be a deeper core emotion in your unconscious that needs to be cleared.

Some of the patterns of behaviours and emotions will have been set in preverbal times, which makes discovering the belief system more challenging. It might be more useful to identify what your unmet needs were. Maybe you were left to cry for hours and no one came, or you learnt that you only got attention when you cried. You might have been angry at being left alone. As you face these deeper emotions and relax through them, you can even clear preverbal struggles. By breathing through what you feel, you may find that you don't even engage with the emotions as you once did because you keep your mind on your breath and not the emotion. You may even find that you can give yourself whatever unmet needs you had in your formative years or know that you can ask for help from the right people. When emotions are triggered, you will know more clearly what you *don't* want, so that you can place more energy and focus on what you *do* want. Starting from a point where you imagine that you have already achieved your goal, by working towards that you start moving into a new reality.

Connecting with and integrating what you have experienced in a more wholesome way can enable you to reconnect with your underlying power, life force or passion for life within you, which may have become buried over the years. The person or situation that harasses you can wake you up to realise a deeper understanding of who you are if the emotional energy is channelled in a constructive way. In that way, you can find meaning to the struggle or suffering you have gone through. If you regularly avoid confrontations, assertiveness training and non-violent communication can be a real benefit if this needs to be addressed.

If you have ever been angry and frustrated as a child and been berated for this, you might have subconsciously decided to not engage with that energy and feel shut down. However, by fearing our inner power, or suppressing anger and frustration, there is a tendency to breathe higher and higher in the chest as we try to escape the uncomfortable feelings in our belly. If sustained, this is more likely to trigger anxiety, panic or asthmatic symptoms. Yawning and feeling sleepy in the presence of an emotionally tense situation can be a sign that there has been an emotional shutdown. By breathing down into your belly and connecting with the power underneath the anxiety or tension in the chest, we can regain connection with our fundamental life force energy.

Although anger is not true power, it is an expression of your life force, just as all your emotions express your life force. Anger can indicate an improvement in our emotional well-being if previously you have felt hopeless or helpless about your health or a situation in your life. When your life force is flowing freely, you experience the pinnacle of well-being through emotions such as love, happiness, joy, harmony, peace and freedom.

Anxiety can occur when we avoid feeling our emotions.[45] This usually creates increasing amounts of internal and external tension in the body. This happens until our system can no longer hold on or we relax. Suddenly, we can have a tidal wave of built-up emotion all release at once. This might explain why some people experience a panic attack when they appear to be relaxing. Avoidance of confronting issues which cause us frustration can also be anxiety provoking. Look at the thought processes or story you might be telling yourself about your situation.

Until you confront your fears, the person or issue will maintain their power over you and can lead to avoidance behaviour.

An Empowering Breath

Different emotions have different styles of breathing. If feeling scared causes you to breathe higher in the chest, breathing down to engage with your power centres in your solar plexus, sacrum and pelvic floor region can be enormously helpful to regain your inner strength. Any breathing should be slow and steady, still in and out through the nose. This can be done whilst you are feeling well or when you are wheezing and feeling depleted. There is a powerful yogic breathing technique called *ujjayi* breathing which helps you to engage with and shift strong emotions and can even help improve your lung function when practised regularly.[46] Learning how to engage with these powerful emotions with your breath will re-energise you in new ways, without needing to reach for a stimulant. When I tried to breathe without wheezing during an attack, I found that ujjayi breathing enabled this to be possible. I will describe the process I went through to completely clear the asthma attack in three minutes in Part Five. Learning the ujjayi breath is a great starting point. From this I developed Dynamic Breath Release, a system of working with and clearing our emotional blocks with the breath.

Ujjayi Breathing

Using ujjayi yogic breathing is a great way to release anger and anxiety with the breath which you can use on your own without needing someone to do a guided meditation with you. Ujjayi breathing is a form of yogic breathing meaning, *to become victorious* or *to gain mastery*. The breath is created by using gentle, sustained pressure from the abdomen to produce a prolonged exhalation through the nose whilst slightly constricting the back of the throat. This should create a sound like waves breaking on the shore. I like to describe breathing in and out through the nose in this way—as ocean breath or dragon breathing. With children (and adults) I get them to pretend they are breathing flames out of their nostrils like a dragon. Imagine you are burning through your unresolved issues as they transform into light. Once the strong emotion has passed, settle into quiet abdominal breathing and allow the heart space to soften.

The Benefits of Ujjayi Breathing

Ujjayi breathing has many benefits. It utilises slow breathing, resulting in increased oxygen absorption.[47] As undertaking this style of breathing requires concentration, it is hard to think about something other than your breath during this activity. It, therefore, helps to bring your awareness into the present moment so that your thoughts become focused on the breath, rather than feeding your emotions with ideas and beliefs that may be untrue. Its effects on the autonomic nervous system are not fully understood, but it does seem to slightly reduce vagal activity which may cause the slight increase in heart rate which has been observed when it has been compared with slow-breathing exercises.[48] This is particularly helpful in the case of an asthma attack as the vagus is usually overactive at this point and the sympathetics have been overworked and have become exhausted. From my personal experience in practice, it appears to have the effect of engaging with the stress response system and may help reduce overactivity in both sympathetic and parasympathetic systems. All we can say is that ujjayi breathing helps to bring the ANS into greater balance.[49]

The ujjayi breath has been shown in studies to help reduce anxiety, depression, calm everyday stress, and stress-related medical conditions.[50] It appears to produce a state of vigilance, a calm alertness which is comparable to the breathing animals do on inspiration when under threat.[51] Over time it may help to establish a better parasympathetic drive,[52] which potentially means the sympathetics don't become overactive to the point of exhaustion, as happens before we have an asthma attack. The prolonged out-breath helps you to release the stress in a manageable way whilst maintaining the underlying relaxation. Yogic breathing studies have demonstrated that it takes around ten weeks of breathing practice to make a difference to respiratory health.[53] Combining this with the breathing retraining exercises, you can notice improvements within the first week. The longer you practise, the more natural it becomes.

STEPS TO MASTERY—Week Two—The Gift in Your Emotions

Most anger is maintained by being uncomfortable with where you find yourself and resisting change. Let go of your fear of the unknown to prevent resistance to the new.

If you do ujjayi breathing whilst feeling angry, you can often resolve the anger and anxiety and feel incredibly energised, which means the person or situation who pushed those anger buttons becomes a gift. Having gratitude for the opportunity to transform your usual reactions into positive responses will enable a more complete healing, rather than remaining unforgiving of the triggers to your emotions. Remember you are emptying your bucket, so you have space for something new to come in.

Having cleared the emotional tension with your breathing you can ask your higher self if you were to respond to your present situation from this place of peace, how would you handle it differently, and what did you previously believe about yourself to feel that way?

What was their behaviour mirroring about how you treated or felt about yourself? Breathe out the old belief and rest in the stillness and peace in the pause. Reclaim your power through your breath, and these old situations can start to become a thing of the past. Whenever you clear something, it is important to fill the space with a new feeling and a more empowering self-belief. For example, you could breathe unconditional love or gratitude into the space where the emotion was. You could even imagine breathing in the opposite of what you have experienced to neutralise the tension, so in place of anger is peace, in the place of fear could be trust. Breathing into the belly helps prevent emotions from stagnating in tension and unconscious holding. Once the emotion has been released, small, reduced breathing helps to quieten us back down into relaxation and rest. Eventually, practising the quiet breathing on a regular basis, many people have found it reduces their emotional volatility, making their emotions more manageable.

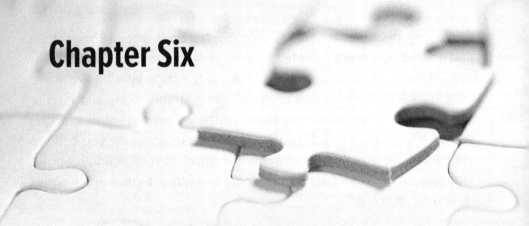

Chapter Six

Seeing the Light

There is nothing either good or bad, but thinking makes it so.

William Shakespeare

Becoming Conscious

As you breathe through old emotional patterns and reduce the amount of unconscious holding, you wake up to new aspects of yourself. You may feel brighter and more energised. Without all the emotional tension your adrenal glands are under less strain, and this will support your healing process.

When you breathe you connect with your spirit. The word spirit means *animating* or *vital principle* and is derived from the Latin word *spiritus*, which means *soul, courage, vigour or breath*. It is related to *spirare* which means *to breathe*. Literally, as we breathe in, we *inspire* or breathe in spirit. The word *psyche* from Greek also pertains to spirit or our combined conscious and unconscious mind. So your spirit lies somewhere between your breath, your thoughts and emotions.

Just as the heart has an energy field one hundred times stronger than that around your head, your body's energy field also expands outwards around you as far as your reach. Your body acts a little bit like a bar magnet. Knowing that you are more than just your body can help to release tension. You can imagine this invisible field holds and supports you as it surrounds you. If you feel depleted emotionally, you can top yourself up by breathing in through the crown of your head and down into your heart. Allow your heart energy to expand further in the pause as you breathe out.

When you breathe in, you can also imagine breathing in through the crown of your head and connecting with your higher self. This is the part of you that is infinitely wise and able to see the bigger picture. If you are feeling lost or confused then accessing this part of your being will enable you to gain a clearer connection. This superconscious part of you is like the antidote to your subconscious programmes. When doing any energy work where you connect upwards, it is important to also ground yourself and connect with the earth.

Letting Go of Control

In order to access more of your life force, it is important to let go of the control formed by your ego self, which forms the personality. The ego self is one of the reasons you may struggle to let go of your emotions. The ego wants to protect itself, and when threatened or challenged will want to resist change. Even though the new reality may be a better one, it clings to the known and fights its demise. As you become willing to let go of old belief systems and ego stories you have about past experiences you will become lighter and more open to changes.

One aspect of changing the story we tell about ourselves is our attachment to a condition. People usually use possessive pronouns about their health conditions. For example, the use of phrases such as, "My asthma," or "I have asthma," is how most people describe the condition. This means our ego self has taken ownership of the illness. Now, although acceptance is a very useful place to be to come to terms with what is, for our body to heal, the ego needs to take a step back to allow these changes. The ego self is like a façade people often put on to cope with life, driven by unconscious emotions. It is often related to unconscious fears such as fear of the unknown, or self-protection, for example.

I used to try exceedingly hard to maintain the illusion that I was in control of my life. I realised what enormous effort this required as actually nothing really was under my control, other than my own actions and reactions to different situations, and even the reactions could be due to unconscious programmes we have inside. By going with the flow rather than forcing things, we can reduce our energy expenditure significantly and life becomes more effortless.

Whilst sat in a traffic jam, late for an appointment, realising that although it would have been easier and probably faster and healthier to have cycled, I was giving myself the illusion that I was the one in control by gripping the steering wheel exceedingly tight and willing the traffic to move forwards. In the mistaken belief that by getting frustrated I could change things, I also feared the unknown of how the person would react to my lateness.

In a moment of clarity, I realised that I was more out of control than ever; all of me was tense. As I let go of making the scheduled appointment, I sat back in my seat realising that there was nothing I could do to change the external reality. I could either arrive at my destination tense and stressed or I could sit back in my seat and just allow the journey to take as long as it needed to.

True patience is not the ability to wait for what we want but to wait with a joyful attitude. As I sat back in my seat, I realised I was relaxed and in control! But the type of control I was experiencing now was a totally new way of understanding it. You are in control only when you let go of control. The traffic then started flowing! When you relax your body, it requires less effort to breathe. The more energy you can free up for healing, the better.

Synchronicity as a Way of Dealing with the Unknown

If you start making changes to your life, stepping into new experiences, you may find yourself having to navigate through the unknown a lot. One of the best ways I have found to cope with this is looking for the synchronicities that arise in our path. These may have been due to intentions we have set and affirmations we have spoken, but could also be part of the rich magic of life.

Whilst navigating my way through my healing journey, I was inspired by *The Celestine Prophecy* which describes following synchronicity as a way of navigating the unknown. Synchronicity is a term created by Carl Jung, founder of analytical psychology. He suggested that rather than life being a series of random events, there is a deeper order that is occurring. Synchronicity describes these meaningful *coincidences*. If someone or something keeps occurring in your reality, it is time to take note and pay attention.

Synchronicity may simply be a self-fulfilling prophecy; when you focus on something, you are more likely to notice it. However, if this does occur, it points to you being a powerful co-creator of your reality. Whatever you pay attention to, you are likely to get more of. Noticing your health improvement is a good practice to start.

Guided Meditation

If you are not used to sitting and meditating on your own in silence, this can be challenging. Rather than being a meditation, it can turn into a massive think-a-thon! Thoughts of to-do lists and whatever current issue is on your mind can often play over and over. If you feel you don't have time to sit and meditate for twenty minutes, you probably need to meditate for an hour. If you find many thoughts arising, you are not trying to stop your mind, simply make friends with it. Focusing on your breathing can help to reduce your mind's activity because it gives your brain one single point of focus and brings you into your body.

Similarly, some people find that when they focus on their breathing, they breathe more or more tension creeps into their breathing patterns. If this has been happening to you, you are not alone. This is why I created guided relaxation sessions for you to work with that don't just focus on your breathing. As you relax during meditation, your breathing slows down anyway. Imagining a scene that is soothing and relaxing to your senses can be a great way to relax. By focusing on the air coming in and going out through your nostrils, you can take yourself into relaxation. This gives the mind one single point of focus rather than many and has the effect of quietening the mind. If you find focusing on your breathing increases anxiety, you might find it helpful to either listen to a guided relaxation or focus your attention on a meditative object such as a candle flame or flower.

In the 1970s Harvard Researchers Howard and Benson showed that oxygen consumption reduced by around 10% during sleep and by 20% whilst in meditation.[54] Carbon dioxide levels also reduced, which meant that cells were not starved of oxygen, suggesting that the body becomes more energy efficient and metabolism slows down during this time in a beneficial way.

Visualisation is a great way to get the mind and body to relax during meditation. It gives the mind something to do. You can be very creative with your visualisations. With your ujjayi breathing, you could imagine the waves crashing on the shore, each wave releasing tension as it breaks on the shore and then retreats. After two to five minutes of ujjayi breathing, you will most likely be able to settle into slow, relaxed, silent breathing and imagine you are now part of a glistening ocean.

Imagining your favourite place of relaxation is another great way to help associate a mental image with a relaxed feeling and your peaceful breathing. Your favourite place of relaxation can be real or imaginary. I always go back to the same imaginary scene of a meadow full of flowers, with a forest to one side and a babbling brook to the other. There is a bridge over the stream to fields beyond and mountains in the distance. I have a healing stone circle that I am safe to sit in and relax inside and receive healing energy as the sun shines down on me. Whatever scene you go to, you should always enter and return the same way. I have a gate that I go through. You could enter by a path or a staircase.

You can also imagine that you are inside a hollow tree with an opening to go inside and become part of the tree. I love to imagine breathing in through the branches in the crown of my head and down and out through the trunk and roots, out through my feet. Then I breathe in through the roots beneath my feet and up and out through the trunk and branches in the top of my head. You can keep these exercises going for a few minutes, adding in the ujjayi breathing to strengthen your experience. If you find yourself in your head during meditation, then this is a very grounding exercise to bring you into your body. Make sure you are still breathing through your nose and into your diaphragm. It is a great way to slow your breathing down and energise yourself.

Emotional Habits

One way you can rob yourself of energy is to maintain emotional habits that drain your energy. Going to bed late, or always working to last-minute deadlines or rushing to make appointments keeps you in a more adrenalised state, eventually leading to exhaustion. Managing your energy levels is a key area to address in the long run so that you can maintain a healthy nervous system. Working too many hours may even be related to an unconscious fear of failure or not feeling good enough. We often only meet with the underlying emotions that feed these ego states when faced with the possibility of not achieving what we set out to realise.

As you make lifestyle changes, you will realise it is far easier to make changes when your subconscious is aligned. Otherwise making these changes becomes a bit like a rider (the conscious mind) trying to turn an elephant (the unconscious) when they both want to go in different directions. If you can get the elephant and the rider to have the same idea, it makes life a lot easier. This will be addressed further in Part Four.

Resolving the Unconscious Death Wish

Sometimes feeling disempowered to act or say something to change a situation, feelings of helplessness or hopelessness may arise rather than feeling anger. Finding yourself in a situation that may have been extremely overwhelming, you may have wished that you weren't there. This is quite common during the teenage years, during the emotional ups and downs of hormonal changes or any abusive situation. This coping mechanism can be helpful at the time but later on in life, when faced with other challenges, there might be a lack of energy to rise to the challenge. This, in effect, is like having a death wish operating at a subconscious level. Until that part of us has a new understanding and drive to live it can sabotage our success and health.

The description of a death wish might seem a bit extreme, but not being able to fully engage with life as it is arising means that part of us isn't present, and may mean that we have only been accessing part of our life force. If you have wished not to be here at any point in the past, even if you embrace life now, that unresolved part of you might rear its head when similar challenges present themselves or simply leave you feeling lethargic for no apparent reason. The part that didn't engage may have left you feeling tired, sleepy or shut down when there is a potential for you to be able to rise to meet a challenge and overcome it.

Having a dialogue with that part of yourself, at whatever age you were when those internal words were spoken, is often helpful. Ask that part of you, "If giving up like this wasn't an option, what would you have to feel instead?" Notice what you feel and use the breath to breathe through these unresolved emotions and then reclaim your power. I ask clients to make a statement out loud to reclaim their power and life force, which adds strength to the transformation. Although the previous words were spoken internally, by intentionally connecting with this part and giving yourself a new, more empowered voice, you can help to heal the split in consciousness and become more whole.

You can now choose to either fully engage or walk away from any situation, in a way that perhaps you couldn't have done as a child. Having this work witnessed is essential to reclaiming your full power. Lethargy and shortness of breath is also a sign of iron deficiency. So getting your iron levels checked would be a good idea.

Alexandra came for breath work and in her case history, described having almost died at birth. During the session she made the connection that her inability to fully engage in her life and have a strong sense of purpose was linked with a pattern that was set up right from her birth when she failed to breathe for some time. Often the way we experience our birth may set up unconscious patterns throughout our lives. Alexandra experienced a strong sense of spiritual connection during her Dynamic Breath Release sessions. Consciously acknowledging that she could experience this in her physical form meant that she could begin to step into her purpose and passion and reap the rewards for this in a way that she had never been able to access before.

A Rainbow Inside

Being human we all have access to the full spectrum of human emotions and qualities. When you recognise an emotion in you that is uncomfortable or challenging, it is good to remember that for pure white light to exist, it is comprised of all the colours of the rainbow. Without red in the spectrum, for example, it would not recombine to form pure white light. By embracing the powerful energies inside you as they arise you can feel fully alive. If you resist them, the drain on the adrenals and nervous system is quite exhausting. Emotions are often fuelled by our thoughts and beliefs about a situation. It is important that you can love yourself enough to validate what you are feeling, and if the emotion doesn't serve you, have the intention of letting it go, allowing your heart energy to be greater than any emotion that surfaces.

You can imagine a rainbow inside you as you breathe in and out. Start with red at the base of your spine, orange at your sacrum, yellow at your solar plexus, green at your heart, blue at your throat, indigo at your brow and white at your crown, connecting you with universal life force energy. Each region is associated with a powerful energy centre, often called chakras in the Indian tradition. They all relate to areas of nerve bundles and hormonal centres that powerfully control your body.

You may feel different emotions are related to different energy centres in your body. You can always imagine spinning the emotion out of your body and breathing the colour into the area to replace it. Each emotion may have a different colour associated with it. You might be able to see it or sense it or simply just imagine what colour it would be. Breathe a new colour of your choice that feels more soothing and relaxing into that area.

Speak Kindly to Yourself

The solar plexus works like an abdominal brain and remembers past emotional experiences from our early childhood, even those that are preverbal. Many emotions arise from this area, and the throat is the part associated with expressing how you feel. Emotions are fuelled by judgements and thoughts arising from the mind. If you hold onto judgements or speak to yourself with criticism and judgement you may feel constricted around the throat and neck. This doesn't help with breathing easily. If you tell yourself you mustn't feel this way or that you should have got over this problem already or that you are not good enough, these can be some of the unspoken words that underlie what we feel. Sometimes coughs can even be related to unspoken words and feelings. You may find that words that you speak internally aren't even yours. They may be words you heard in your younger years. In meditation ask whose voice you are really hearing.

The greatest journey you can ever take is from your solar plexus to your heart and from your head to your heart. Here you find your true centre. The challenges you face and overcome on the way will increase the depth of your love and peace. By naming the emotion that you feel you can reduce the intensity of your experience.[55]

It is important to approach any self-development work with self-compassion. Beating ourselves up for not being good enough, or falling short of our idea of being perfect, only creates further tension and resistance to change. I have taken that path too many times! Finding an internal voice that is kind can take some practice, especially if you have been prone to self-judgement and criticism. One of the most healing things you can do for yourself is to acknowledge the reaction within you as being the best you can be at that time. Self-acceptance fuels the desire for greater love and self-compassion and personal growth. The more compassionate you feel towards yourself, the greater acceptance and understanding you have for others. You can make choices that nurture you and your health. Don't look back on what might have been; see the abundance of who you are right now.

If you are in the habit of ritually giving yourself an internal beating, such as having feelings of not being good enough or punishing yourself through overworking or criticising how you look or even how you feel, you may well be in need of a compassionate angel.

Having experienced the death of her brother, Sally found that imagining a compassionate angel speak to her at times when she was unable to find loving words to say to herself, was a powerful way of stopping this self-critical voice and replacing it with a nurturing, caring voice. There may be a special place or image that works as a reminder of your compassionate angel so that you can start giving yourself some loving encouragement. It could be a statue or a photograph pinned on your mirror of someone you respect, who could say something kind to you as you look in the mirror. Think about how you would speak kindly to a friend, and if you have no one to witness your situation, then speak kindly to yourself as you look into the mirror. Beam love into your eyes and allow your heart to receive it. You will be able to give more to others when you like more aspects of yourself.

By simply accepting life as it is in this moment, without judgement or preference for something else, the part of you that is prone to struggle and strive feels so supported. The reduction in tension enables the fear reactions to simply wind down. Acceptance doesn't mean it will always be this way. It's just how it is in this moment, and in the next moment, change is possible. Once you have faced your fears and your emotions you have a new space for joy to bubble up inside enabling you to live life from this freedom.

The Moment of Choice

There is a split second between a thought arising and the reaction in your body. If you catch this space between the thought and the feeling arising, you can choose to let go in your body rather than engage with it. This is where your breath pause can be useful. Your emotions can pass through you, without attachment to them. There is no right or wrong way to feel about something. How you feel is due to your past experience. If you can identify the story of your past experience and be willing to let go of the story and the emotion through the breath, then it creates the possibility for change.

Many of our reactions are responses to beliefs we have developed through our early childhood or earlier adult experiences. We cannot change our past, but we can change how we respond to our past memories and present-day situations which may resonate with our previous experiences.

Emotions are fed by the stories we tell ourselves about them. This rumination only seeks to strengthen our experience of them.[56] The emotion will fill the gap between where you find yourself and where you would like to be. If you can identify the story you are telling yourself and you are willing to let it go, you will start to reduce the emotional intensity. By accepting where you are you will also bring about greater peace of mind. You might be able to identify your story by noticing what you don't want so that you are clearer about what you would like. It may be that underlying the emotion and not having your needs met, is a story of not feeling good enough or worthy of what you desire. It may be that you don't value yourself enough and this is being mirrored externally. Breathing through the emotion and then surrendering in the pause at the end of the out-breath, you can be curious to see what your new reality could be.

Once the uncomfortable emotion has cleared, there is a space for something new. You can then imagine breathing in a feeling of already having your emotional needs met, maybe even breathing in what it feels like to be enough. Having released the old tensions and breathed in an empowering feeling, whatever the external reality, you will have closed the gap. Being hooked into externals to make us happy will never bring true lasting happiness. It is only when we feel contentment on the inside that we can experience a real depth of happiness, which will be translated into you experiencing positive emotional health. Breathing into the feeling of already having what you would like brings freedom. Whether you have it or whether you don't, it is the same.

If you imagine your emotions are like a tuning fork of a particular frequency, ping a tuning fork and it will resonate. Bring a second tuning fork of the same note next to the first, and it will start to vibrate without being touched. Once you shift your emotional frequency, by letting go of past hurts, and breathe into your open-hearted feelings, you are more likely to be a resonant match to positive experiences showing up in your reality. This is known as the Law of Attraction. One of the fastest ways of changing your emotional state is to listen to your favourite music or sing.

Healing the Past

As a child I loved the film *Back to the Future*. They travel back to the past in a time machine. Changing the past created changes when then returned to the present. In some situations we may wish we had a time machine. Although you can't change what has happened, you can change how you feel about it through guided meditation. You can only come to peace and forgiveness with a situation when you have released the stored emotional hurt and pain around the issue. Then the present situation can change in the ways you *respond* to things, rather than *reacting* from old patterns.

The hot air balloon meditation is a great way of combining emotional healing of the past with breathing techniques that will enable you to access the consciousness of your higher self—clearing your old patterns. By integrating the past and the present, you can release your attachment to old issues so that you can have greater freedom in the present. You can float back at a safe distance to an earlier time and drop a rope ladder to the part of you from an old memory. This younger part of you can then see the situation from a new perspective and connect with your adult wisdom. Recovering yourself from the past, you can stand right behind this younger part of yourself, to give support, so that you don't feel alone, and then travel forwards in time to the present, getting a sense of how things can be and how easy your breathing is. You can even move further forwards into the future to feel how these changes transform your reality. If you have come to a place where you are happy with where you are now, it is easier to come to peace with the past, as it made you who you are today.

When you resolve an old emotional issue, it sometimes feels like nothing has happened although there is often a lightness that wasn't there before. You might intrinsically feel the same. However, when faced with a similar issue again, rather than reacting automatically from old emotions you notice how effortlessly you respond to it from your new perspective. Once you have faced your fears and resolved them this enables a new reality in the present, opening new avenues for the future.

Use whatever situation has triggered your emotional response as a gift to bring you greater self-awareness. You can either react habitually, as you have done previously with these situations, or you can break the habit by responding differently. By identifying what you are feeling in your body and where you feel it, and focusing only on the feeling, you give your mind a task other than focusing on the story which prevents the emotion being fed and allows both the story and the emotion to release. Emotions can last under two to three minutes if you really embrace what you feel and allow it to disperse with the out-breath. During our Dynamic Breath Release workshops, we use guided imagery as a healing modality to help you heal past hurts and discover your full potential.

STEPS TO MASTERY—Week Two—Hot-Air Balloon Meditation

Self-enquiry is a great way to bring to your consciousness ways in which you might have been unkind to yourself. For example, how have you criticised or judged parts of your body / behaviours for not being good enough? Take a few moments each day this week to send appreciation to those parts which you have judged and send acceptance to those parts of you that you may have rejected. Place a hand on your heart and a hand on any other area of your body that needs some kindness and imagine you can breathe light into that part to integrate it. You may also reflect on ways in which you can give yourself more space and time.

Use the guided meditations to help heal past hurts so that you can move forwards with greater ease. Notice what happens when you feel different emotions. Scan your body and notice any areas of contraction. Where does the emotion arise? Once you can name what you are feeling and where you feel it, become aware of what happens to your breathing as you notice these feelings.

Don't try to change what you feel or try to fix it, simply welcome the feeling, but don't wallow in it. If the emotion is the wave, it is the power of the ocean behind the wave that you are after. Your connection to your essence, your life force is to be found in the still point at the end of the out-breath.

If you are on your own and a strong emotion arises, look into your eyes in a mirror and beam love to yourself through your eyes. It will stop you getting lost in the emotion and prevent you from feeling alone. Allow yourself to feel what you are feeling, until the wave passes. Expand into your compassion for yourself and others in your heart. Know that there is an energy field larger than you, or your ego, holding you to enable your healing transformation. If you need help from your higher self, you only have to ask. If you need to transform significant emotional traumas from the past, find support from a practitioner, such as an experienced hypnotherapist. It is important to have your transformation witnessed. Give your body time to heal; your support of this process is cumulative.

Sit down and focus on slow, relaxed breathing three times a day for 15-20 minutes. You can listen to the guided meditations, or you can begin the breathing retraining from Part Five. If you feel your emotional life is in good order and you already have a healthy diet, begin your breathing retraining. If you still have further lifestyle changes to make, don't try to do everything at once, pace yourself. If emotions arise later on, you can always come back to these pages.

When it comes to emotions, you don't have to take responsibility for other people. You only have to be responsible for yourself. Seeing others as being capable for themselves, will prevent a lot of unnecessary worry. If your emotions are continuously like a roller coaster, it could simply be related to adrenal fatigue. Addressing this with mindful breathing meditation and supportive nutrition is a significant help. Giving yourself time to rest is also invaluable.

Remember, when you register this copy of your book you will be able to access lots of guided meditations and other resources linked to each section.

PART THREE—

NUTRITION

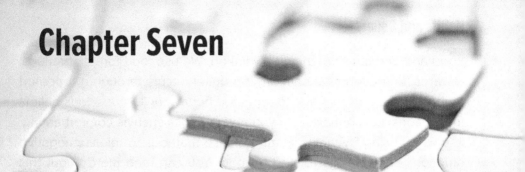

Chapter Seven

Food to Support Your Healing

The doctor of the future will give no medication,

but will interest his patients in the care of the human frame,

diet and in the cause and prevention of disease.

Thomas Edison

There are many different ways that nutrition can directly and indirectly affect your breathing, both for the better and worse. These can range from food intolerances and allergy, which create more inflammation in your body and increased mucus production narrowing the airways and making nose breathing difficult, to mechanical aspects such as abdominal bloating, making it challenging to breathe into your abdomen. Food intolerances can also heighten anxiety states, possibly because the stress reaction it causes increases breathing rate which activates the limbic system in the emotional brain. Some foods even stimulate the fight-or-flight nervous system thereby adding to the physiological or body stress that our organs experience. The habits and use of food in a social context can also influence your food choices. If the wrong food choices can make you worse, getting it right can also be a massive support for your recovery.

Habits and Beliefs

Food and emotions are incredibly linked. We use food for celebrations, rewards, and even as a comfort. If a belief occurs through a repeated thought, a habit occurs due to repeated behaviour. Unconscious beliefs fuel unconscious behaviour. If you notice habits such as comfort eating, it is worth using Dynamic Breath Release methods to release negative emotions and feelings related to food. You can read more about this in Part Five. If you weren't to go for your favourite snack or reach for that extra biscuit, what would you feel? Are you tired, thirsty or feeling emotional?

Creating healthy habits with food relies on us also being happy and mindful of our choices. Cutting foods out altogether can often create cravings and further tension. Finding healthy natural alternatives to your favourite foods is a good starting point. Correct nutrition is crucial for natural health and healing. Once your body has recovered, you won't have to be as strict with your food choices, but having a basic healthy eating framework to come back to is helpful. You might also want to write a list of non-food related treats, such as a soak in the bath or time to read a book, so that you can give yourself a reward for anything you achieve during your day. Food doesn't always have to be the main reward system.

Natural Food and Foodless Food

Fast food has been associated with an increased risk of developing asthma.[57] Fast food is often devoid of the micronutrients essential for health. The nutrients in natural foods provide energy for your body's healing and repair processes. If you are eating foods that take more energy to break down and create an excess of waste products for your body to deal with, this will take energy from your body's healing processes and reduce your healing ability. *It is your inherent tissue intelligence which does the healing; the food simply energises the processes occurring within your system.* Even when overloaded, your body is still acting intelligently, doing the best it can with the current situation. The illness you experience is simply its coping mechanism or adaptation to maintain as near normal functioning throughout the rest of the body. What you bring into your body may enhance or diminish this natural intelligence. A diet high in unprocessed plant-based foods full of micronutrients is essential for good natural health. It is not necessarily what you cut out, but what you consume that is most important.

Inflammation

One of the main components of asthma is the inflammatory response. Inflammation is needed by the body to help heal and repair tissues. If your body becomes out of balance, inflammation may become chronic and adaptive symptoms arise, in an attempt to heal or maintain health. Often this creates a vicious cycle of further stress due to discomfort and then further overbreathing due to pain or constriction of airways. Inflammation is produced by a cascade of different chemicals within the body, including histamine, leukotrienes, and prostaglandins. Histamines are released from mast cells which are part of your body's immune system. High histamine levels and allergies are linked.

At the top of your fight-or-flight chain, in the brain, the hypothalamus releases Corticotropin-Releasing Hormone (CRH) in response to stress. This chemical messenger tells the pituitary gland it needs to release ACTH (Adrenocorticotropic Hormone). The Release of ACTH into the bloodstream activates your adrenal glands to produce adrenaline and cortisol. CRH is known to destabilise mast cells so that they release their histamine,[58] giving the many different symptoms of inflammation across many different organ systems of, including asthma and eczema and allergies. Put simply, histamine is released from mast cells when your body is stressed.

Normally the cortisol released would act as an anti-inflammatory. However, at the point of adrenal gland exhaustion, CRH might still be released in an attempt to maintain the stress response but instead causes chronic inflammation to set in as the mast cells are activated instead. Your body is assuming you have experienced a trauma that needs repair, from the prolonged fight-or-flight activity. During raised cortisol levels your body's main focus isn't on the organs of elimination so there will be an underlying increase in metabolic waste, which can create a fertile breeding ground for bacteria. When you reduce your breathing and relax, you may find that the eliminatory organs actually start to clear a backlog of waste, known in naturopathic (natural healing) principles as a healing crisis.

Allergy and Breathing

Hyperventilation not only raises histamine levels but many allergy sufferers are hyperventilators and many allergic reactions also cause hyperventilation.[59] This creates a feedback loop that requires changing. Although in theory by improving your breathing you should be able to improve your digestion, in order to break the cycle, it is often necessary to cut out foods that you are allergic or intolerant to, in order to help reduce the inflammation and further stress to your body. In time your intolerances may diminish, but you will need to have eliminated foods for at least three to six months to let your system calm down. In the case of severe allergy, I would never recommend reintroducing them as this can be life-threatening. It is interesting that the medical treatment is to have an adrenaline (epinephrine) EpiPen to inject in such cases. If the adrenals had not become fatigued in the first place would so many allergies exist?

Inflammatory Mediators

There are two other inflammatory chemicals that play a key role in lung inflammation; leukotrienes and prostaglandins. Arachidonic acid is a precursor to leukotrienes and prostaglandin production, which both promote inflammation.[60] Excess amounts of arachidonic acid can, therefore, fuel inflammation and aggravate asthma.[61] The main sources of arachidonic acid come from animal products in the diet, such as meat, eggs, dairy and fish.

If you remove these from your diet, you can help to break the inflammatory cycle.[62] In fact, in a huge study in Australia with over 156,000 people analysed, those with asthma and or hay fever had diets higher in meat, poultry and seafood intake. In another study of over 765 students in South America, intake of fish once a month was shown to be protective against asthma due to the protective effects of the omega-three oils reducing inflammation, but the high histamine content could increase the risk of hives if over consumed.

Fish is only high histamine if it is not fresh, it is the bacteria growth that increases the histamine content. The quality of the fish consumed is also to be considered. Farmed fish, which includes organic fish is not in its natural habit, but in large pens, and fed with artificial feed products. Non-organic farmed fish will have antibiotic treatments added to the water which will affect the quality of the fish. Wild, deep sea fish is probably the healthiest for your body. Eating fish once or twice a week can be helpful to maintain B12 levels. The faster it is frozen after being caught, the lower the histamine levels will be. If it smells fishy, avoid it.

There are different ways of dealing with chronic inflammation. The slow nose breathing exercises over time will help to reduce the stress response which, will reduce the histamine levels. Cutting back on animal products can make a huge difference to the levels of inflammation experienced, for some. Cutting out foods that directly stimulate the stress response are also best avoided. This is because artificially stimulating your stress response may give temporary relief, but leads to further exhaustion over time. This includes removing chemical additives and stimulants and foods that you might be intolerant to.

Caffeine Stimulates the Fight-or-Flight Response

Caffeine increases cortisol levels, [63,64] stimulates an increased respiratory rate, [65] and increases anxiety and panic attacks. [66,67] If you manage to keep your breathing rate slow after having caffeine, it has been shown to increase vagal activity. [68] In the case of an asthma attack, this is not wise at all. Needless to say, caffeine interferes with the ANS. Trying to regain natural balance is impossible whilst using stimulants. Stimulation may give a short-term gain but creates longer-term pain and problems. Caffeine uses tomorrow's energy today. It is like using an overdraft.

As both tea and coffee cause dehydration—they are diuretics and histamine are released in response to dehydration—a better response would be to have a glass of water. Chocolate has also been associated anecdotally in the Buteyko Method with reduced control pause times and hyperventilation and should be avoided. As caffeine causes problems with insomnia,[69] it can reduce your body's ability to get the deep rest that it needs in order to restore itself. Stimulating yourself back to health eventually leads to exhaustion.

Bloating

The prolonged sympathetic dominance which is associated with long-term hyperventilation and overbreathing is associated with bloating.[70] This not only makes abdominal breathing more difficult but can further worsen the effects of stress and poor digestion. As soon as you can consciously start breathing down into your abdomen more regularly, you will have an improvement in your digestive health. You could be eating all the right foods, but if they are not properly being digested or absorbed because of the stress levels in your system, it will not be as helpful as it could be.

Worrying is another reason that blood is diverted away from the gut and sent to the brain as you think through situations. There is only enough blood in the body to do one thing at a time efficiently. You can digest, think or exercise. Try combining them and the blood supply may not be sufficient. You can fit all the blood in the body into the gut if all the blood vessels are fully dilated. Leaving exercise until at least two hours after having eaten will support the digestive process.

Is What You are Eating Making You Ill?

Everyone's food needs are slightly different. There is no one set diet that will suit all people. There are however some general health principles that have stood the test of time for many years and foods that you should definitely avoid if you want to encourage natural healing. There may be some foods that enhance your health and some that diminish it.

Sometimes when you start eating more healthily, the body can have a healing crisis as it starts to eliminate the backlog of waste stored in the tissues. This is often when the greatest healing is happening. This is why when you eat healthier food you can sometimes initially feel worse before feeling better. Relaxing through this and trusting the process rather than fearing it is the best approach. Know that your body is taking the best possible care of you. If the changes result in a worsening of symptoms over time, there could be something that is still irritating your system. You can feel a bit flat for the first week when cutting something out of your diet and headaches can occur too. These should pass within the week. Drink plenty of water. You should be starting to feel an improvement after two weeks. If not, get some extra nutritional support.

Allergy and Food Intolerance

Allergy UK estimates that 45% of British adults have some kind of food intolerance.[71] Food intolerance is different to an allergy. If you have a food allergy, you will likely know within a couple of minutes of eating the food that your body is reacting to it, with symptoms such as nausea and vomiting, throat constriction, and a puffy face. This is known as an anaphylactic reaction due to an immune reaction involving immunoglobulin E (IgE) and histamine release.

A food intolerance blood test checks for food reactions to immunoglobulin G (IgG) which is a much lesser response, and usually comes on over several hours and can continue over two to three days. An IgG blood test, checks for the immune reaction to food protein particles that manage to pass through a compromised mucous membrane in the intestines and enters the bloodstream. Here the body tries to remove them through the IgG immune response creating a widespread inflammation in the body.

There are other foods that your body can also be sensitive to. All chemical additives should be avoided. A reaction to these is a sign your body is healthy enough to spot non-natural substances and try to clear them quickly. If your body has a lack of enzymes in the digestive tract, lactose in milk can also increase bloating, flatulence, infantile colic, abdominal pain and diarrhoea,[72] or constipation.[73] Histamine-containing foods such strawberries, tomatoes, some cheese, wine and nuts, can also cause a reaction in the gut causing nausea or vomiting, diarrhoea, rashes or flushing, headaches and a runny nose.[74] If you have food intolerances, some people even find it causes their moods and emotions to be more volatile. Cutting down on high histamine foods can be helpful alongside meditation and mindful breathing.

There are also bio-resonance hair tests that are available to test your intolerance, which in my experience tend to give similar information to the blood test and may pick up on other chemical areas of sensitivity. This is a less expensive option than the blood test. The blood test cannot be done if you are taking steroid medication as it can affect the results. The hair test can be taken even if you have excluded foods already.

Symptoms of Food Intolerance

A food intolerance reaction can have the same symptoms as an allergic reaction, but is usually less immediate but still causes an excessive histamine release, which can lead to swollen lips, urticaria (hives), vomiting and diarrhoea, a runny nose, headaches, and difficulty breathing.[75] Muscle aches, joint pain, and tiredness on waking that isn't relieved during the day are common symptoms. [76] In the digestive system itself, indigestion, reflux or heartburn, colic, bloating and diarrhoea are common.[77] When your body is inflamed, it will often store the waste products of inflammation in fat tissue, so weight gain is also common. Inflammation and an immune reaction in the intestines can heighten other immune responses in the rest of the body. Although abdominal symptoms of bloating, diarrhoea and constipation may occur, there isn't always an obvious response in the digestive system immediately. The following diagram shows some of the symptoms of food sensitivity other than the digestive disturbances which can occur.

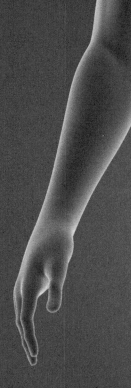

The Central Nervous System

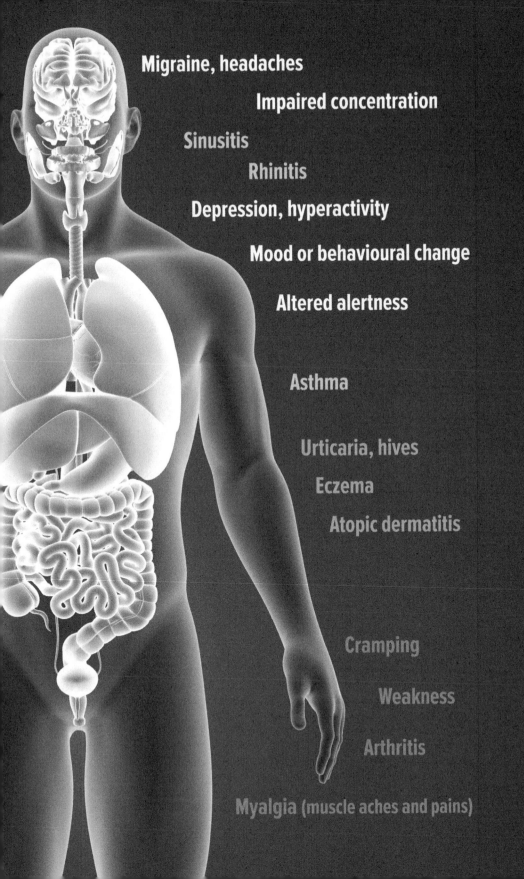

Migraine, headaches

Impaired concentration

Sinusitis

Rhinitis

Depression, hyperactivity

Mood or behavioural change

Altered alertness

Asthma

Urticaria, hives

Eczema

Atopic dermatitis

Cramping

Weakness

Arthritis

Myalgia (muscle aches and pains)

Although osteoarthritis is usually related to wear and tear or trauma in joints, patients that I have seen in practice commonly report cutting out dairy and wheat products reduces their painful symptoms. Rheumatoid arthritis, an autoimmune condition, has been associated with "leaky gut" syndrome also known as increased intestinal permeability and altered gut bacteria, known as dysbiosis.[78] Rheumatoid arthritis often coincides with a reduction in Bifidobacterium, [79] a naturally occurring probiotic bacteria in the gut. It has been shown that mast cells which produce histamine can also create leaky gut problems and chronic stress also increases intestinal permeability.[80]

The Cause of Food Intolerance

Food intolerance and over-consumption of food is a growing issue amongst many people and a factor which can maintain chronic health conditions. Blood supply is often diverted away from the digestive tract when the body is stressed, and the diaphragm doesn't engage to give the intestines their usual massage. This means that food can rot and ferment rather than digest. The gut not only absorbs some of the breakdown products of rotting food, but it leaves a fertile breeding ground for bacteria and even yeast to proliferate. As the yeast proliferates, it can attack the lining of the small intestines and make them semi-permeable to larger proteins such as gluten, known as leaky gut syndrome or small intestine permeability.

It doesn't have to be yeast causing the inflammation. Studies have shown that leaky gut can even be caused without infection by long-term stress or after trauma and surgery.[81,82] If the intestine wall is inflamed it doesn't produce digestive enzymes in the same way, so, for example, gluten causing inflammation in the intestines can also reduce production of the digestive enzyme lactase. This, in turn, can mean that the lactose in milk isn't digested as readily. I have had many patients with arthritis and asthma cut out wheat and dairy produce and sugar to find that their asthmatic and arthritic symptoms have significantly reduced. Reducing the gut inflammation reduces the inflammation body wide. The symptoms in the body can occur up to three days after the food has been eaten, making identification of the irritating food difficult.

Identifying Food Intolerance

I have found experienced kinesiologists can muscle test for food intolerance fairly accurately. It is a very useful tool in ascertaining which foods cause your body to weaken. In my experience, it can often produce results similar to that obtained by a food intolerance blood test. In some areas, a blood test will not show up all the foods your body is intolerant to, as it is testing an immune reaction to proteins in the food. For example, it doesn't test for lactose intolerance, but would test for milk protein intolerance. There can be other substances within the food you eat that challenge the body that might not show up. You will have to have eaten the food several times at least three months before the test for it to register if there was a reaction.

There is also hair sample analysis, which works through bio-resonance techniques which can detect intolerance to many different foods and non-foods, which is a less invasive option. Depending on hair length it provides a longer period of health to study. Having compared hair analysis with the IgG blood test, the hair analysis gave similar results and was more affordable. If you suspect an allergy, this can be tested with an IgE blood test available from your doctor.

It is interesting to note that if you eat a food that you are intolerant or allergic to, within twenty minutes of eating the food your control pause will often be significantly reduced. This can be a simple method you use at home to see how you respond to a particular type of food. Testing companies suggest cutting foods out for three months if intolerance has shown up. Research has shown it can take up to six months for immune reactions to clear from the blood.[83] I initially cut foods out for six weeks as it seemed more achievable and I felt better within that timeframe, so I stuck with it. Why would I go back to feeling pain?

Why Six Weeks?

Many of the processes in the body take six weeks. This is because the cells in the liver, bones and muscles all live for six weeks. Six weeks from breaking a bone, as long as it is set correctly, the bone will have mended. In six weeks' time, all the cells in the liver have turned over one cell generation.

Whatever you put into your body over this six-week period will help inform the health of the next generation of cells. If you have had a strain, injury or illness you want to put the healthiest foods into your body to encourage the best repair process possible. Similarly, when you are recovering from illness, this is the time to put only the most natural foods into your body to regain your full vitality. Continuing on even when you are well again is ideal.

My Experience of Food Intolerance

If I hadn't experienced the pain and health problems associated with food intolerance first hand, I don't think I would have appreciated how much of a difference to your health you can make by eating the right foods for your body. By my early twenties, I was waking with burning pain in my feet, knees and lower back, had abdominal bloating and frequent interstitial cystitis. My face and chest were still covered with acne and my hair was very thin, a sign of excess prostaglandin production and hormonal imbalance. This was on top of allergic asthma. Somehow, I hadn't connected what I was feeling in my body with food, because I believed I ate a pretty healthy diet and didn't particularly have any digestive problems other than a known allergy to peanuts (which I avoided) and mild constipation. I didn't have abdominal pain directly after eating. However, sometimes even foods that we might consider healthy are maintaining chronic health problems.

Having seen a Homeopath who kinesiology-muscle-tested me for food intolerance, I cut out dairy, yeast, chocolate and sugar for six weeks. Six weeks later, I was waking without pain. I tried reintroducing those foods one at a time to notice how my body reacted. The skin problems or joint aches returned, so I kept them out. Almost twenty years later I have stuck to keeping these foods out of my diet wherever possible and have no joint aches and pains, my skin cleared up, and I am in better health than I was in my twenties. Having since included mindful breathing practice into my repertoire, keeping my control pause high, I find I can eat some of those foods occasionally without any major repercussions, although sugar, yeast and cow's milk are not essential to good health.

Many years later I took a food intolerance blood test. Yeast and dairy showed up as foods causing an immune reaction. It was interesting that the kinesiology results were verified through clinical laboratory testing. I began to take steps towards taking more responsibility for my own health. For a self-confessed cheese-aholic, this was no mean feat. We often crave the foods we are intolerant to. During my naturopathic training, I studied this area in greater depth to be able to gain a greater understanding of how this issue can affect your health, which has enabled me to help guide others through this challenging area.

Does Dairy Increase Mucus?

Dairy consumption hasn't directly been linked with asthma, although some people will have asthmatic symptoms after consuming dairy produce.[84] Dairy consumption has been shown to increase inflammation in the gut,[85] which could, in turn, lead to increased mucus production throughout the body. In my own clinical experience, sugar and refined carbohydrates will also predispose to increased mucus production.

Review Your Diet

It is good to start with removing food additives, colourants and artificial preservatives, refined foods and stimulants from your diet. You can replace cow's milk with organic oat milk and rice milk, but in the fullness of time, it is cheaper and healthier to learn how to make almond milk and oat milk yourself. Many of the pre-made milk alternatives contain many artificial additives. *Rude Health* and *Organic Oatly* are exceptions. Food replacement products are far from healthy foods. Gluten-free foods often use flour made from products which are still refined and processed, lacking fibre they will rapidly release sugars into the system and resemble glue to the intestines. A whole-food plant, based diet is the best way to improve health.

You might want to begin by reviewing what you eat. If your main consumption of dairy is on cereal for breakfast, there are very few cereals on the market that don't have an added sweetener or sugar of some type. The original muesli was mainly grated apple and not the dry mix that we have packaged on our supermarket shelves today.

Not just Eliminating but Supplementing

Breakfast could consist of a fresh vegetable juice made with a juice extractor. Increasing the amount of fresh produce in your diet will increase the micronutrients, both minerals and vitamins that you take in. Juicing makes the living nutrients more readily available and easier to absorb. It is a more natural and healthier alternative to supplementation. Plant nutrients usually occur in a balance which encourages their uptake in our body unlike the dead chemical compounds found in tablet supplements. A glass of freshly made carrot juice has many healing properties and can help improve immune system function and repair DNA. [86]

If you don't have access to a juice extractor, then a bowl of watermelon is a lovely way to start the day, full of lycopene as well as the many other vitamins and minerals it contains, which have health-enhancing effects. Lycopene is known for its anti-inflammatory properties.

Nutrition is Key, not Just Elimination

When eliminating unnatural and processed foods, it is important to get the right dietary advice specific to your needs. Removing food groups might cause you to miss out on other vital nutrients contained within them, which could lead to a deficiency which can also cause health problems. If you are vegetarian and you cut out dairy and eggs, you have removed your source of vitamin B12, which is essential for producing healthy red blood cells and the production of myelin which protects your nerves and prevents neurological illness.

Vitamins are known to have a protective effect on the immune system and reduce mast cell activity.[87] For example, vitamins C, D and E are all shown to have an effect on strengthening the immune system, as are the B vitamins, especially vitamin B6. [88] Vitamin B6 is found in animal products and grains, which, if removed from your diet, is also available in chickpeas and millet. Vitamin E is found in almonds, spinach, sweet potato, avocado, sunflower seeds, plant oils and butternut squash. As vitamin D is produced with UVB exposure, having some time in the sun each day is likely to boost your health which is not always so easy in the winter months and why vitamin D deficiency is increasing in the UK, especially with the use of sun creams. The ideal daily exposure of your body is twenty minutes if you are of Caucasian origin and forty minutes if you are of African or Asian origin.

Vitamin C is required to also help make adrenaline and supports the adrenal glands. Vitamin C has been shown to reduce elevated cortisol levels more quickly after an episode of acute stress[89] and is also required to aid iron absorption which is needed for healthy red blood cells to carry oxygen around your body. Vitamin C is more than just its chemical formula ascorbic acid. It is a wide array of bioflavonoids that can only really be found fully in their plant-based form.

Oranges and lemons, although high in vitamin C, can pose problems for some, as they can produce more mucus and in some cases can make asthma and arthritic conditions worse. It is best to obtain your vitamin C from dark green leafy vegetables and if you tolerate peppers and berries these are other sources high in vitamin C. If you don't tolerate oxalates well, rocket, also known as arugula, is a good source of low oxalate greens. Cooking destroys vitamin C. In an experiment to determine which method caused least destruction of vitamin C between microwaving, boiling, stir-frying or steaming for five minutes, boiling was the worst; reducing content by 38% alongside microwaving and stir-frying. Steaming showed not much difference to raw broccoli content.

Food for Thought

By removing the foods that your body is intolerant to, the stress on your digestive and immune systems will be reduced. This enables energy to be directed towards healing and repair, improving your health in ways you might not even begin to be able to imagine. For me, it was like I had had a hole in my boat and energy had been taken up bailing the water out, rather than mending the hole and being able to sail forwards. My body had learnt to *tolerate* the dairy, yeast, sugar and chocolate by compensating with skin eruptions, joint aches and pains and hair loss and frequent bouts of cystitis. This was a high price to pay for a modern diet and way of living. All of these remain at bay when I keep my diet clean and maintain my relaxation.

STEPS TO MASTERY—Week Three—Identify Food Intolerances

Keep up the breathing exercises each morning and use the control pause measure to establish whether a type of food is causing you to hyperventilate. A lower control pause around twenty minutes after you have eaten a food will usually indicate the food has potentially caused a strain on your system. Cut out any foods that are definitely causing a reaction for you. If in doubt, have a blood test, hair analysis or find an experienced kinesiologist to test you. Make sure that, whatever foods you cut out, you find other health-producing foods to replace those nutrients. Focus your attention on health rather than trying to overcome leaky gut or an infection. My focus during my own recovery was always on health improvement rather than fighting disease.

Invest in a juice extractor to be able to juice vegetables and supplement your nutrient intake. It is a great way to start the day. Have time out in the fresh air every day to exercise and move your body.

Writing a food diary of what you have eaten and how you feel before and after eating can be useful to find out whether your triggers are particular foods or particular stresses. There is a basic elimination diet with foods that are low-sensitivity that you can do for two weeks. After two weeks, adding new foods every third day will give you a chance to notice how your system responds to the challenge. If you react, keep them out longer-term. This should be done under the supervision of an experienced nutritionist so that you don't end up missing major nutrients from your diet. This can be a time-consuming process and may be easier to have a test.

Chapter Eight

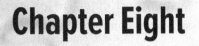

Improving your Health

Be moderate in order to taste the joys of life in abundance.

Epicurus

Patience Is a Virtue

It usually takes a tenth of the time it has taken to become ill to heal and recover. For example, with unhealthy living over a decade and a chronic health condition, it will take a year to give your body the constitutional support it requires to recover, depending on the severity and amount of changes required. Some people with incredible vitality and strong genetic inheritance can turn things around more quickly. It all depends on how chronic and long-standing the condition is and how many changes you are willing to make.

The Gut and Your Health

As around 70-80% of your immune system is based in your intestines,[90] having the right balance of beneficial bacteria in your intestines, known as probiotics, helps aid your immune system and digestive process. It also means that in order to strengthen your immune system, your digestive health needs to be top priority.

Along with the lungs, your digestive tract is a tube open to the outside world. Given the density of immune tissue in your intestines, it follows that health improvements to your immune system arise from restoring gut health. Having the right nutrition is the foundation of your health improvement. From there everything else can follow.

If your gut flora has become imbalanced over time from unhealthy or stressful living, yeast overgrowth can occur in the intestines, the most common being the yeast *candida albicans*. Candida occurs naturally in around 70% of people.[91,92] It is only when it overgrows that it becomes a problem. It can result in IBS (irritable bowel syndrome), including bloating, cramping and gas. If you also suffer from oral thrush, vaginal thrush (cottage-cheese-like discharge) and itching, sore throats, jock itch, or itchy burning eyes or itchy ears, it may well be due to candida overgrowth. However, candida is not the cause of your problems. The *cause* is the overindulgence of sugar, refined starches, stress or medication—causing toxicity and a reduced immune function. Excesses and toxicity exhaust your system, known as enervation. This reduces the expression of vitality. Killing the candida with medication does little to address the underlying health problems behind its proliferation.

Many of today's food products include sugar. We eat more sugar now than ever before. Over-consumption of refined sugar, fruit, gluten-containing grains and dairy, leads to gut flora imbalance. Yeast thrives on sugar in the forms of glucose, sucrose, fructose (fruit sugar) and lactose (milk sugar). When sugars are readily available in the intestines, they are more likely to encourage an overgrowth. However, fruit sugars are bound within cells and with fibre, so there is a much slower release of the fructose. Overripe and dried fruit may well aggravate some severe cases of candida or gut dysbiosis—an imbalanced gut bacterial flora. Fruit juice, even if freshly squeezed can also be a problem.

Choosing a diet to reduce excess sugar, I would recommend avoiding refined sugar, excess fruit consumption through fruit juices and too many dried fruits, refined wheat, dairy, white rice, white pasta, white flour products and alcohol. If you are yeast-sensitive and candida infections occur frequently, then yeast should also be avoided. Many of the symptoms of candida are similar to the symptoms of leaky gut. So they are probably not all caused by candida but by the increased permeability of the gut affecting different organ systems, and the ways in which your body will try to compensate or be overwhelmed by that. Artificial sweeteners should also be avoided not only for the toxic effects as they are broken down, but they could confuse your body when it thinks something sweet is coming and it isn't which could possibly cause more sugar cravings. It is also worth noting that refined starch, for example, white flour, white rice and white pasta and even crisps and chips, all rapidly break down into sugar. You will probably be aware that none of them are health foods.

Medication and the Gut

Although all medication to some degree will upset the natural balance of bacteria in the gut, the birth control pill,[93] antibiotics,[94,95] steroids[96] and a more neutral pH[97] in the digestive system, which can occur with overuse of antacids, are known contributing factors. Anti-inflammatories are also known to destroy the gut mucosa, making the intestines more permeable and can lead to cell death in the digestive tract, and intestinal bleeding.[98,99] As the environment changes within the digestive tract, it makes the overgrowth of yeast, known as candidiasis, more likely. This can trigger you to crave products such as sugar or bread, as the yeast in the gut requires sugars to ferment, as with making bread or brewing beer, thus maintaining the imbalance. Chlorine and fluoride in tap water can destroy the healthy bacteria in your gut which can also create an imbalance. Drink clean, filtered water only.

Candida has been shown to produce ethanol,[100] acetaldehyde[101] and ammonia[102] as its by-products, which can lead to brain fog and mood alteration, poisoning the body and causing further ill health. If ever there were was a reason to give up excess sugar and refined starch, which rapidly breaks down into sugar, this would be it.

Yeast colonisation of the intestinal mucosa is known to trigger allergic reactions.[103] Asthma has long been known to be triggered by candida albicans infection.[104] The overgrowth creates an immune reaction which, on top of asthma, can also cause eczema[105] and is associated with inflammatory conditions. The growth of candida albicans was promoted in the intestines of mice given antibiotic treatment. These mice became sensitised to allergens, such as proteins and mould spores, causing hypersensitivity of the pulmonary airways[106] and reactive inflammation.[107] Mice without the candida infection showed no signs of allergic airway response to allergens.[108]

Candida starts out life as a round, single-cell yeast, but it can develop into a fungal form with excess sugar. The fungus has hyphae or tendrils which can penetrate the intestine wall and cause hyperpermeability of the mucosa.[109] There is a recognised association between the reduced barrier function of the intestinal mucosa, known as leaky gut, disturbances in the gut microflora and atopic disease[110] (allergies). Leaky gut allows proteins, such as gluten, bacteria and undigested particles, to enter the bloodstream causing an immune reaction and inflammation. The immune reaction to these food particles is described as food intolerance.

Inflammation is the immune system's direct response to this food intolerance and the breakdown in the protective lining of the gut. This can cause more widespread symptoms of inflammation throughout the body. Left unchecked, leaky gut syndrome and the immune reaction from food intolerance can, in turn, lead to autoimmune conditions.[111] With waste overloading the tissues of the body our natural healing mechanisms become overactive, using inflammation as its main response to attempt to clear the waste. These inflammatory symptoms are simply the body's best attempt at restoring health.

Leaky gut may sound quite alarming, and it can cause significant challenges to the maintenance of good health. However, it should be noted that we are talking about microscopic leakage of particles. It is not large-scale leakage which would arise due to a ruptured intestine or perforated bowel, a much more serious and acute condition. Leaky gut is more likely to cause long-term chronic ill health. This causes huge physiological stress on the body and gives our eliminatory organs, such as the liver and kidneys, even more work to do. This leads to further tiredness and ill health as our additional cellular waste won't get eliminated as effectively.

As asthma treatment often involves steroid medication, which affects gut flora and can lead to candida infection,[112] and candida can lead to asthmatic symptoms, this becomes a cyclical problem. It is important though that you NEVER suddenly drop steroid medication. Steroids are prescribed when the body is exhausted and unable to produce enough natural cortisol to keep up with the stressful demands placed on it. It is important to boost your health and vitality before making any changes under the supervision of your registered medical doctor.

Symptoms of Candidiasis

The following list of symptoms is commonly attributed to the end result of candida overgrowth.[113]

- Fatigue
- Weakness
- Feeling of being hung-over
- Muscle & joint aches
- Headaches
- Gastrointestinal disturbances—diarrhoea, constipation, nausea
- Bloating after eating
- Psychological disturbances—depression, anxiety, irritability, mood swings
- Cognitive dysfunction—brain fog, poor memory, lack of concentration, difficulty concentrating or focusing
- Recurrent vaginitis, vaginal or rectal itching
- Urinary tract infections
- Menstrual disturbances and Infertility
- Loss of sex drive
- Allergies, including shortness of breath and chest tightness
- Skin irritations/rashes/acne/itching
- Fungal nail infections or athlete's foot

- Sugar cravings
- Recurrent throat/ear infections, itchy ears
- Hypoglycaemia and sugar or bread cravings

Hormones and Candida

Hormonal imbalance and candida go together. The birth control pill actually increases candida infections. Candida contains oestrogen receptor sites which utilise this hormone for its growth.[114] It is possible that candida may also create hormonal imbalance and has coincided with adrenal and thyroid deficiency, as well as being present in diabetes and kidney problems and even in lung fibrosis.[115] Removing the causative factors of candida may help address the hormonal imbalance along with dietary changes. Normally oestrogen and progesterone balance each other out. When cortisol is high after ovulation, it is associated with lower levels of progesterone,[116] producing a relative oestrogen dominance.

Oestrogen dominance can cause mood swings, hot sweats and hair loss, water retention, trouble sleeping, and breast swelling and tenderness, fibrous cysts in the breasts and irregular periods. When oestrogen is dominant, it can feed the candida yeast and make it more virulent. Excess adipose (fat) tissue in the body also produces extra oestrogen which can also contribute to feeding the candida, and excess weight will often result from high stress and an excess of high carb, high sugar and low fibre meals, which also directly feeds yeast.

Initially, eliminating the sugar and refined foods can cause a worsening of symptoms as the die-off of candida can also release acetaldehyde and phenols which can be quite toxic to the liver and kidneys. The symptoms of candida are related to toxaemia and toxicity in the body. There is no way of determining toxicity levels other than through the severity of symptoms, how long-standing they have been and how quickly you recover. There are stool and blood tests that can identify candida overgrowth, which nutritionists can perform.

Not all of the symptoms of IBS can be attributed to candida overgrowth.[117] This means that we cannot blame all the symptoms we experience on yeast. As we mentioned before, Corticotrophic Releasing Hormone can make the gut lining more sensitive and permeable.[118]

If you are having digestive and health difficulties, then it is important to make the necessary dietary and lifestyle changes to reduce your stress levels. The approach to cleansing your diet should both reduce candida and bacterial overgrowth too, as high carb and sugar diets will affect both. The cleanse is also a low-inflammatory diet which should help to reduce the inflammation throughout your body. Many health conditions are related to inflammation and if you have a low-inflammatory diet, you will be supporting your body back to health.

Allergies from Being Too Clean

In 1989 Professor David Strachan proposed the *hygiene hypothesis*, which suggests that the lack of exposure to germs in childhood and fewer childhood illnesses are to blame for the rise in allergies. Studies with animals have given support for the hygiene hypothesis.[119] Being too clean and overuse of antibacterials will have contributed to a decline in our healthy bacterial flora. In the next few years as bacteria become even more antibiotic resistant, we could be forced to move back to a more natural approach to healthcare and healing.

Focus on Health, not Disease

So now you know where you don't want to be, it's time to start moving forwards towards health. The most exciting thing to realise about these symptoms is that if they can be caused by dietary and lifestyle choices, they can also be reversed by dietary and lifestyle changes. You have great power to restore your health.

Having a practitioner with the confidence to guide you through this process is an enormous help to enable you to face challenges in areas where you might be in the dark. Eventually learning to listen to your own inner guidance is essential. Then you can begin transforming your life.

Peter came for breathing training and found that by doing the Buteyko exercises his candida infection cleared up and he was not craving sugar any more. His energy levels also increased.

The Health Benefits of Probiotics

It is amazing to realise that having the right probiotic healthy bacteria, that naturally colonise the gut, could improve your mood. A study with mice given probiotics showed changes in brain chemistry linked to improved mood. The link between the gut and the brain chemistry was found to be through the vagus nerve.[120] If the vagus is stimulated in the gut in the right way, then the lungs are more likely to function healthily too as they share this common nerve pathway.

Probiotics have been shown to reduce inflammation in the body,[121] along with having a beneficial effect on allergy in children.[122] They can even have a beneficial effect on more chronic inflammatory bowel disease such as ulcerative colitis when used over a two-month period. [123]

After a month of nutritional cleansing and healing has occurred it is time to add in some probiotics. If you think you are suffering from leaky gut, I would not recommend taking probiotics until you have had at least 4-6 weeks off the main inflammatory-causing foods; wheat, dairy, eggs, yeast, sugar, caffeine, red meat and food additives or artificial sweeteners. If you have had a course of medication, I would always recommend taking an additional probiotic supplement for up to three months afterwards to enhance the gut flora, but only after having done a digestive cleanse.

In the long term, it is useful to add in probiotic foods to your daily diet. This could be sauerkraut (fermented cabbage) or kefir (fermented milk using a kefir starter culture). Some people with histamine sensitivity may find these difficult to process. Plain natural probiotic yoghurts are fine for those who do not have a dairy intolerance. For some, they can be digested more easily as the probiotics have digested the lactose. I would avoid shop bought probiotic yoghurts that have added sugar or artificial sweeteners in them. These provide little value as a health food and often don't have enough bacteria to make it through the stomach acid and into the intestines. The milk has been heat-treated and pasteurised; this affects the proteins and fats within the product, which changes the way the body assimilates them.

Goats' and sheep's milk is more similar to human milk so probiotic yoghurt made from these milks can be more digestible than cow's milk. If you can find a local source of organic milk, you can buy kefir starter cultures online to make your own kefir. Alternatively, some raw sauerkraut made from cabbage and Himalayan salt or unrefined sea salt is the best option. The souring or fermenting of the cabbage produces beneficial bacteria which will help digest your greens and salads, breaking down the cell walls so you can extract the micronutrient mineral goodness.

Kale is also a useful addition during this cleansing process as the molybdenum it contains is good for neutralising the acetaldehyde the candida produces as they die off,[124] as is parsley. Occasionally people feel worse before they feel better when they have more probiotics. The probiotics literally crowd out the bad bacteria and yeast and cause their demise. The body then clears out the dead bacterial waste products. This is an active process that doesn't happen as effectively if you just kill the bacteria or yeast with medication, as the body has not mounted an active elimination process.

It is so vitally important when faced with many symptoms that we remember not to become overly focused on the disease. Whatever you focus your energy and attention on you will get more of. Many people can diagnose or name diseases. To look for health in your body, as a good alternative health practitioner would do, and cultivate this is a good skill to develop. Health is not merely the absence of symptoms. It cannot be found in a tablet or pill or supplement, it comes from within. It arises from following the laws of nature, from not overindulging, by living within your means, and allowing yourself enough rest and play, and breathing effectively.

STEPS TO MASTERY—Week Three

Although there have been some time frames provided here, your body works at its own rate, and you cannot force change. Give yourself time to heal and commit to the journey. It can take a year or more in some cases.

It is vitally important to sit down whilst you are eating and rest for 20-30 minutes after eating to aid your digestive process. Chewing your food thoroughly before swallowing is essential too. If the food is broken down more, it will give less work for your internal organs and you will receive more nutrients from the food you have eaten. You will notice that if you chew with your mouth closed and breathe only through your nose, you will also swallow less air which leads to less bloating and gas. They may seem like small changes, but simple changes can make a big difference over time.

Eating healthily and still not noticing an improvement? Symbolically, if you have unclear boundaries on your energy and are over-giving to others and people pleasing, the internal body and digestive system could mirror the lack of boundaries. If your body is under excessive tension or if you have had an emotional shock, then whatever foods you eat will not be tolerated or digested well. Therefore, clearing your emotional tension can be the most important focus for your health. Take your problems for a long walk in the countryside or a stomp in the park to gain a fresh perspective. If symptoms are progressively worsening, seek professional help and support from your doctor or experienced nutritionist or naturopath.

Be Aware...If you are still suffering from lots of bloating and gas, you might also consider investigating the FODMAP diet,[125] which lists foods containing carbohydrates that are known to cause increased fermentation and bloating and loose stools.[126] You can use the low FODMAP diet as a baseline and then add in another type of food every couple of days as a challenge to see how you respond to it. As beans and pulses are high FODMAP, try soaking them overnight and sprouting them over 3-4 days watering them daily. Bean sprouts are a tasty addition to your salad and may cause fewer reactions as sprouting activates their natural enzymes making them more digestible. You might be able to include small amounts of higher FODMAP foods in your diet without too much of a problem. Again, remembering to chew your food well, relaxing whilst you are eating and having the right probiotic balance can also help with their digestion.

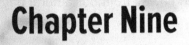

Chapter Nine

A Natural Path

Life is a series of natural and spontaneous changes.

Don't resist them—that only creates sorrow.

Let reality be reality.

Let things flow naturally forward in whatever way they like.

Lao Tzu

A Way Back to Health

How far have you moved from your natural roots? The way many people live today is completely unnatural compared to our caveman or primate ancestors, and yet our internal physiology has hardly changed. To enable the intelligence of natural healing to flourish we need to be living as close to nature as possible. Nature doesn't make mistakes with health, we make choices that cause a strain to our nature. The more choices we have, the greater the possibility of moving away from our natural path, which can lead to dis-ease.

A natural approach to health utilises natural methods to support the healing process, such as nutrition, fasting, hydrotherapy, compressing, massage and exercise, baths and sunlight. These simple *Nature Cure* methods give people the possibility to access their best possible health and learn how to maintain it.

What is Nature Cure?

Nature Cure is a branch of naturopathic practice looking at natural healing, without the use of herbs or supplements and sees the body as having the inherent intelligence within the system to be able to bring about healing, if we respond wisely. By living as naturally as we can and supporting the body through the healing process using compressing, fasting and a plant-based whole-food diet, we can trust our body's inherent intelligence.

The word *cure* comes from the Latin *cura*, which means *management, administration, care, concern* and *charge*. Nature Cure is, therefore, natural care. If you are looking for a natural cure for dis-ease, you are really looking to discover what the correct natural care is. There are many different ways people show care, not all of them natural. What orthodox medicine describes as cure is often suppression which inevitably leads to the expression of the dis-ease occurring in a different form, known as a side effect. Finding the cause of the dis-ease within your body, and resolving this, helps to clear it at its source. Natural health requires living naturally, which also means living in harmony with our planet and our surroundings. If any part of the whole is out of balance, then full health cannot exist.

Finding the Cure

Caring for yourself is a way of life. Care isn't something you just do when you are unwell. Some people become a little frustrated when they realise that the only cure is right living and right action. Some people may say eating a healthy diet isn't a cure if it means their symptoms return when they don't eat healthily.

You wouldn't just vacuum your carpet or service your car once and then expect that it would be fine forever more. Living in a human body is a skill that, with practice, we can improve with age. The symptoms your body expresses are the body's way of attempting to remove the causes of dis-ease.

It is important that you energise your system with vital living and health-giving foods. The more refined, processed or cooked a food is, the more it destroys its vitalising enzymes, vitamins and minerals which are vital for health. For many years I was puzzled as to why, even though I was eating healthy foods, I still had allergic responses, until I discovered the Buteyko Method, and started to retrain my breathing patterns, which you can learn about more in Part Five. In my own life and in my practice experience, making lifestyle changes to support the breathing practice is the best way to make a lasting improvement to your health. I believe the excess acid produced by the breakdown of processed foods could make us breathe more rapidly just to expel the extra acid from our body. Having lots of raw and fresh foods will mean that your breathing is automatically slower.

Increasing your Nutrient Intake

The old adage, "You are what you eat," is not necessarily always true. You are not just what you eat, you are what you absorb. You might fill yourself full of health-producing food, but if your body is so depleted it cannot absorb the nutrients, then having additional ways to relax your body with the breath will also help encourage recovery.

If your body is not in a state able to accept natural foods and digest them easily, juicing is one way to enable your body to uptake the micronutrients really easily. Because there is no fibre to digest, the juice and its minerals and vitamins will be absorbed straight into the body. However, it is important to remember that when juicing it should be vegetables that are mainly juiced with the addition of one apple.

It is not advisable to drink fruit juices as this will overload the body with fruit sugars. Without the fibre to buffer it, the sugars get absorbed too rapidly, which could affect your system adversely. It is also important to remember not to buy your juices, as they will often have been heat-treated which destroys the natural enzymes and denatures the vitamins, and that is what your body benefits from with fresh juice.

Fruit Juice and Immune Reactions

Whilst I was studying with my grandfather I was amazed to notice that if I drank freshly pressed apple juice in the presence of his cat, the wheeziness would start almost immediately. One day when I went to my grandfather's house, instead of juice I had water. The wheezing didn't start until I ate food. I realised that there was a strong connection between what we eat and drink and how our lungs and immune system respond. I was amazed at how instantaneously the reaction occurred. I now know that sugar and even fruit sugars can weaken the immune system. If you were to eat as many apples in one sitting as it takes to make a glass of juice, you might well struggle to eat them in one sitting. One of my patients managed to relieve his wheezing after exercise simply by hydrating effectively.

Hydration

Hydration is a fundamental part of maintaining health. Many people talk about drinking eight glasses of water per day, however, in Nature Cure practice this may be excessive and can lead to tissue congestion, increased activity for the kidneys and a loss of minerals, as the urine will take minerals with it. If any fluid is over consumed there can be a rise in blood pressure as the extra liquid increases the blood volume. Increased volume causes increased pressure. If the kidneys are overloaded and become exhausted the result will be increased blood pressure. If you have been used to having several drinks of tea, coffee or soft drinks each day, start replacing them with filtered water.

It is better to have foods that have a high water content that will enable a gradual release of mineral-rich water into our body, such as lettuce and cucumber, greens and fruit in their raw form. Four glasses of water per day are adequate if you are eating a plant-based diet with raw foods in a moderate climate; maybe more in a hotter climate or with exertion. Gorillas seldom drink water. If 60% of every meal is fruit, salad and vegetables you will obtain two litres of water per day easily.

Tea reduces iron uptake and, over time, the tissues harden from the tannins they contain. Tannin is used to harden leather. If you are thirsty, drink spring water or at least filtered tap water. Some areas have fluoridated water which is toxic to the thyroid gland and isn't removed by water filtration or boiling. Try infusing some freshly grated ginger into warm water or some freshly picked peppermint leaves for a refreshing warm drink. Both ginger[127] and peppermint[128] have been shown to reduce allergic responses.

What Happens with Dehydration?

If we consume excess table salt, the concentration of sodium outside the cells is greater than inside the cells, which draws water out of the cells into the interstitial fluid; the fluid between the cells. This can create dehydrated cells and waterlogged tissues. When the cells are dehydrated, they don't function properly.

Drinking caffeinated drinks, such as tea and coffee, as well as alcohol, all have a diuretic effect on the body which means we lose more water than we are taking with the liquid, which inevitably leads to dehydration. When we become dehydrated our mast cells produce more histamine. Histamine is released with dehydration because it attracts water molecules, which try to hold onto the fluid. The increased water and histamine in our tissues causes them to become enlarged or inflamed, which causes pain in our tissues or, in people who are susceptible, the narrowing of the airways in the lungs, and difficulty breathing. This inflammatory response is our body's cry for water. As you know, histamine is overproduced in people who suffer from allergies and many inflammatory conditions. If the body is properly hydrated and relaxed, then there is no need for excess histamine production. Some believe that intracellular water in raw plant food is easier to absorb.

Acid-Alkali Balance

The body must maintain an almost neutral but slightly alkaline blood of pH 7.3-7.4 for all the cellular reactions in the body to work. If it goes above or below this, then systems stop functioning properly. There are buffering systems in place to maintain this. The fastest acting of these systems is achieved through breathing. The most important part of the buffering system related to breathing and for the main regulation of pH for fluid outside of the cells is the carbonic acid-bicarbonate buffering system. As carbon dioxide joins to water, it forms carbonic acid. If the blood becomes too acidic, our breathing rate increases and we breathe out more CO_2.

Acidity in the body increases our breathing rate. We literally blow out the acid as we breathe out carbon dioxide. This means that hyperventilation may have initially been triggered by an excessively acid diet and then the body just got used to breathing that fast or must continue at this rate to maintain the normal blood pH. Slowing the breathing down will mean that any extra acid will have to find a different route out of the body, which could create symptoms of heightened elimination, which is why people with kidney problems shouldn't do the slow-breathing exercises.

The kidneys are the slower acting buffering system, eliminating excess acid or alkali through urine production—maintaining an equilibrium, known as homeostasis. Minerals in your body and in your diet also help in this buffering system. Minerals such as potassium, calcium, magnesium and sodium can all attach to bicarbonate. As the acid levels outside of the cells rise, potassium, which normally has a higher concentration inside the cell, moves out to maintain a more neutral pH.[129] This can also lead to muscle aches and pains. Potassium is found in all fresh fruits and vegetables and is readily absorbed through the gut.

Even though meat would have been part of the Palaeolithic diet, it would never have been consumed with as great a frequency as it is today. Reducing the acid load on your system is one way of rapidly improving your health. An overly acidic body arises from the accumulation of waste products from cellular activity, such as lactic and uric acid, including the breakdown of stress hormones which also increases the acidic state. Much of the grain and protein-based food we eat also breaks down into acid residues.

Pure water has a neutral pH of 7. The scale means that for each integer decrease in pH the acidity is increased ten times. This means pH6 is ten times more acidic than water, pH5 is one hundred times more acidic. Most fizzy drinks are pH3, which means that they are 10,000 times more acidic than water. Putting highly acidic foods and drinks into your body makes the buffering system work very hard to maintain health. Most plant-based wholefoods have more alkalising residues due to their mineral content. The body can lose a lot of stomach acid very rapidly by repeatedly vomiting and put the body into a relatively alkaline state. During illness, this may be one reason why we vomit, as a way of regulating our neutral pH and reducing our acid load.

When we slow our breathing down, the body may need to find other routes out for the extra acid waste, which can trigger an eliminatory event. This is quite normal and will pass. Having a whole-food plant-based diet will help with extra minerals which also help buffer the blood pH and stop the body having to dump the excess acid into our tissues making them ache. If you have ever had a stitch, which is the lactic acid formed in muscles with intense anaerobic exercise, you will know that acid in your tissues causes pain. In the main, most plant foods, not including grains, will break down into alkaline residues in the body which help to neutralise our acid waste such as lactic and uric acid.

Increase Your Greens

When most people are asked to increase their fruit and veg, they will increase their fruit intake, but will not increase their greens. Greens are one of the foods which are often forgotten. Having a salad meal every day is crucial to improving your energy levels and health. It is also important initially to be vigilant to which foods and drinks cause a reaction until you get to know your body better. Often increasing your greens will increase the peristalsis or wave-like motion that moves your food through your digestive tract. This should eventually adapt. It is highly beneficial to enable the clearing of any retained waste in the digestive tract which is often reabsorbed into the body. Some people are oxalate sensitive, and this is contained in greens. Be aware of keeping oxalate foods low if so. As mentioned previously, rocket can be a good source of low oxalate greens for your salad.

Finding and Removing the Cause

When you start to make positive changes your body wakes up, like having a spring clean. The symptoms experienced are often a result of your tissue intelligence having enough vitality to throw off the toxic waste that has accumulated in your system. When you add more energy to a system, everything gets louder, the good and the bad. If we actively work to eliminate what we no longer need, then we can have an overall improvement in health.

The healing process can often be uncomfortable. It is only once the repair and elimination of the waste products has occurred that you start to feel the benefit of improved health and well-being. If you have suffered from a chronic health condition for many years, the body uses the acute illness or healing crisis as a way of healing and restoring health, both physically and emotionally. It is vitally important to support this process and allow the body the elimination it requires. After all, if there is waste coming out, there is no point pushing it back in or suppressing it. The more rapid the detoxification, the more severe the symptoms of elimination. The less we resist and the more we enable the process, the easier it is.

What are the Symptoms of Healing?

Symptoms of a healing crisis and detox can be any acute illness. Acute refers to a condition with sudden onset which can change rapidly. It can be anything from an increase in mucus production and sweating to a headache, shakiness, dizziness or light-headedness, increase in frequency and odour of bowel or bladder elimination, or a rash. In extreme cases, a rise in temperature or fever and general aches and pains can occur. A fever helps to burn through the waste along with destroying bacteria or viruses feeding on it. This is why it is not advisable to suppress a fever.

A chronic condition simply means a health situation that has been more long-standing. The body tries to heal from chronic conditions through acute illness. However, the acute stage must be managed effectively, or there will be a worsening of the chronic condition. As the body eliminates excess waste, these symptoms should all improve. As you begin to come out of the healing crisis, you will generally start to feel an improvement in your mental and physical well-being. If there is a general worsening of symptoms, this can point towards a disease crisis rather than a healing crisis. It is worth consulting a qualified health professional, familiar with this type of healing to support you during this process.

Sometimes the acute process seems to be more intense than we can tolerate. If you are eating a plant-based diet and want to slow down the elimination, some brown rice is useful to reduce the intensity of detoxification. Having simple, natural methods, such as hydrotherapy, to help ease the acute presentation is always helpful, as fear of the symptoms can also heighten the experience of pain. Compressing is one form of hydrotherapy which can be helpful to aid elimination.

As your body is energised by fresh, natural foods, it enables your system to throw out the old waste. However, if you feel worse and stay worse, this is not a healing crisis, this is the body trying to make us aware that something is not quite right and calling on us to make changes.

When you improve your natural nutrition, eating closest to your natural roots, in most cases, will improve health regardless of the condition. The lightness of the food you eat will allow you to feel lighter in your emotional self too.

Supporting the Elimination

As you change your lifestyle, the waste products begin to be eliminated from the body. With an increase in cellular waste excretion, this can result in many of the symptoms associated with a healing crisis. It may take weeks or months of healthy living to develop a healing crisis, as it will only occur if the body has enough vitality to throw out extra waste. If you develop a fever during the crisis, have bed rest and water only for three to four days. If you can't manage three days on water or if you are taking medication, then, when your fever reduces and your appetite returns, you can reintroduce some vegetable juice. Carrot juice is one of the most soothing on our digestive system and cleansing to our blood. In fact, it has been used for the treatment of chronic disease for decades, and one study has shown that carrot juice extract can even kill leukaemia cells and inhibit their progression.[130]

Melon is also very easily digested. Giving your digestive system a rest means more of your body's energy can be directed to healing and less to the digestive effort. When you lose your appetite and fast, this is known as physiological fasting. Elective fasting can be done when you are relatively well, to give your system a rest, but physiological fasting often produces the most powerful results as the body is already in a state of heightened elimination. You slowly reintroduce food once your appetite returns.

Hydrotherapy

Whilst your body is healing it is great to feel you are actively engaged in the process and supporting your own health. Hydrotherapy is the application of hot or cold water to the body through bathing, showering, or with a cloth, applied to various parts of the body to encourage circulation. It is important to know that it should not be applied in conjunction with medication as it can lead to undesirable effects as the kidneys can be overloaded if medication is used at the same time.

The Waist Compress

To support elimination through the kidneys and intestines, the use of a waist compress at night or whilst in bed is helpful. Wet a strip of cotton or linen in cold water wrapped once around the abdomen, just a bit narrower than a scarf. A dry fleece or woollen scarf is then wrapped on top of the linen and safety pinned in place. The cold water stimulates a lasting warm response which brings more blood to the organs of elimination. The compress must warm up within five minutes of putting it on. If it doesn't warm up, remove it and put on warm clothes. You can try again 20-30 minutes later or another night. The waist compress can be worn two to three nights in a row or alternate nights. During a fever, it will help draw the blood away from the head and can be worn repeatedly until the fever breaks.

Having gone through my whole childhood and adult life without medication for illness, the compress is our main form of medicine. As a child I didn't relish wearing one; however, it often helped to soothe a tummy ache or a high temperature. In fact, it was a test of how unwell we actually felt as to whether we wanted to wear it or not! After becoming a naturopath and applying it with patients in my clinic with inflamed lower backs, I could see the rapid recovery they made even if their condition had become static. Even patients in my clinic diagnosed with prolapsed discs have benefitted from pain relief from the waist compress.

Alternating hot and cold flannels on the abdomen are also useful to ease congestion and discomfort in both the abdomen and lower extremity.

Cold Shower or Splash

To encourage your lymphatic system and blood circulation you can finish your shower off with a cold shower or splash, followed by a vigorous rub with a rough towel to encourage a warm pink reaction on the skin. This helps improve the oxygenation of skin and muscles and assists with the drainage of waste products. Cold showering must be carried out in a warm room, with warm clothes to hand to wrap up afterwards. Place your arms, legs, abdomen and back under the cold water for 2-5 seconds whilst rubbing towards your heart. Remember to rub your lower back to stimulate your kidneys. The idea is not to make you cold but to try to stimulate the body into a warm reaction to improve the circulatory system.

Alternatively, fill the bath with about 10cm of cold water. Kneel in the bathtub and splash thirty cold splashes—ten onto your abdomen, ten between your legs and ten onto your lower back. As the cold water contacts the skin the tissues will contract. Between the splashes, the muscles relax. Splashing is better than showering because it creates a pumping action in the tissues which will improve the circulation in the areas applied such as the lower back and internal organs. It helps to tone the tissues. Remember, vigorous rubbing with a rough towel towards the heart is best after a cold splash to stimulate the blood circulation and lymph drainage afterwards. Your aim is to create a warm pink reaction on the skin. Holding your abdominal muscles in whilst rubbing, tones your tummy. It is a great way to wake yourself out of depression or sleepiness on a morning, and much healthier than a caffeine kick-start!

If your feet hurt, then simply walking in cold water and giving them a vigorous rub dry is helpful. Lie on your back with your legs up the wall for twenty minutes once a week to aid the drainage from your legs.

If you feel wheezy or tight-chested, it is also helpful to apply a cold flannel between your shoulder blades and wait for it to warm up, to ease the breathing, and then go to bed and rest.

Maintaining the Change

Once you have come through your healing crisis, there is a critical shift that needs to take place after you have followed guidance from someone on nutritional changes, from following them to deciding within yourself what path you will follow. You are free to choose health in each moment. Sometimes there is grief for the life we are letting go of, but there should be so many positives from the increase in vitality that these outweigh the old habits you have let go of. If you are tempted by something, give yourself permission to have it and then pause for a moment before taking any action. Sometimes the very act of giving yourself permission to have something means that you can choose not to and instead choose health. If temptation wins, still give yourself full permission, as guilt will worsen the strain on your body, then make sure that you have lovely fresh food in the following days. Instead of chips, I have sweet potato wedges, dry roasted, and I substituted chocolate with Medjool dates, which were just as much of a treat, and not as easy to overindulge in. Write your non-food treat list and stick it on a kitchen cupboard or treat yourself to a delicious vegetable juice.

STEPS TO MASTERY—Week Three—Dealing with a Healing Crisis

Watch the videos on supporting the healing crisis, with practical demonstrations for compressing and cold splashing.

Ask yourself, "How can I honour my body with the food I eat today to improve my health?"

Once you have a new healthful nutritional routine, just get on with enjoying the delicious fresh food and don't worry about it. Once in good health, there is an 80:20 rule. Eat 80% for health and you choose what you do with the 20%—which might equate to two or three meals in a week. Whilst you are still recovering, you might need to be mindful of your nutrition for up to a year. Let go of guilt and other emotions in relation to food and give yourself nurturing comfort. Reward and support yourself in ways that are unrelated to food. Give yourself permission to make a choice either way. This will give you greater freedom to choose the best action in each moment.

Try and eat organic wherever possible to reduce your exposure to chemicals. If you can't afford to buy everything organic, then just buy the foods that are known as the *dirty dozen*, the foods with the highest chemical residues, in their organic form. Apples are often top of that list.

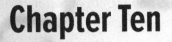

Chapter Ten

Healing with Raw Food and Fasting

Fasting is the first principle of medicine;

fast and see the strength of the spirit reveal itself.

Rumi

Regaining Trust in the Body

If you have had health challenges, you will understand that sometimes the trust in your body has to be rebuilt. Having already recovered from one knee injury, I managed to inflame both knees to twice their normal size on a 260-mile bicycle ride from York to Snowdonia over 3½ days. In hindsight, a bit more training might have helped, as would a lighter load. But having returned home by train, two weeks later my knees were still stiff walking downstairs on a morning. Now, the link to breathing might seem tenuous here, but not many people have only one health problem, there are often different challenges throughout our lives. The recovery from this knee incident was to teach me even more about nutritional healing and trusting the healing power of my body and natural food.

My grandfather, Leslie Harrison, now a retired naturopath or Nature Cure practitioner, suggested that I have two weeks on a raw food diet. I wasn't exactly sure how this would make a difference as I already had a largely plant-based diet, with two raw food meals each day. I knew that the gut referred pain to the knees, and had cut out the foods I had been found intolerant to, but not gluten. My evening meal was a vegetarian savoury dish with greens and vegetables. I had also taken to making spelt and rye soda bread, both containing gluten. I decided to give the raw food a try. The next day I walked downstairs without limping. I wondered whether this was just the natural progression of the condition, so that evening I ate a cooked meal and the following day I walked downstairs and felt stiff again. So again I had another raw food day, and the following day I felt much easier. How was that possible? The inflammation had significantly reduced.

Once you have seen how your body can heal one area, you then just need to trust that, with the right support, your body can also heal the lungs. The first time you ever manage to go through an asthmatic event without having to reach for your inhaler is a momentous day. You can always have it to hand, so you know it is there in case you need it, but it is enormously freeing to learn how to work with the breath, rather than fight it. When you find yourself just breathing easily in all situations, you have truly found your freedom.

Ten years ago, in the final year of naturopathic training, I went to stay in Australia with Dr John Fielder, osteopath and naturopath and president of our naturopathic society, the ISRN (The Incorporated Society of Registered Naturopaths). He has now lived on a raw food diet for around fifty years in the tropics, which had enabled him to overcome asthma, along with arthritis, migraine and a fractured spine, when a car he was working on landed on him. I was so inspired by his story of healing that I decided to undertake a year on raw food. I knew that a raw food diet would be easier to undertake in the warm climate of the tropics and ripe, nutrient-dense, tropical fruits would be more accessible in Australia than they would be back home in the UK.

In the run-up to my year on raw food, I kept dreaming about buying only watermelon and pineapple from the supermarket. The organic vegi-box and a trip to our local natural food store would provide me with everything else I needed. My subconscious was programming me for a year on raw food, like a mental rehearsal or self-hypnosis. This meant that there was no struggle between conscious and unconscious choices. All of me chose to do it.

Watermelon is highly cleansing and with its high lycopene content is a natural anti-inflammatory. Pineapple is great at clearing mucus. Both foods are highly beneficial for those with congested breathing and mucus overproduction. A word of caution here, pineapple should never be eaten after a fast, as it contains protease, an enzyme which digests protein. This is great for tenderising meat, but not so good if the stomach is delicate or if you have a stomach ulcer. You don't want your internal organs tenderising.

After three months of completely raw food, I added in cooked eggs, brown rice and quinoa and jacket sweet potatoes, to compensate for the colder climate of the UK and make sure I was receiving enough B12 with the eggs. Within a couple of months, I was amazed to find I could go to family and friends homes with animals without having any breathing reaction. I was delighted.

Raw Food Reduces Inflammation

Further evidence for the benefits of raw foods was demonstrated in a study carried out by Dr Paul Kouchakoff M.D. from the Institute of Clinical Chemistry in Lausanne, Switzerland, in 1930.[131] Leukocytosis is a medical term referring to an increase of white blood cells in the body, known to increase inflammation. This usually happens when an infection or an immune system challenge occurs. Kouchakoff revealed that a process known as digestive leucocytosis occurs when we eat cooked food but not when we eat raw food. This means that the body responds to cooked food as though there is a low-grade immune response. If this happens continually when we eat, it could be weakening the immune system.

In my case, it certainly explained the rapid improvement when I switched to raw food for a couple of weeks whilst my inflamed knees were recovering. Kouchakoff did, however, find that as long as you eat over 50% of each meal as raw food, digestive leucocytosis was not as apparent.

Only a couple of weeks into eating raw food, I noticed my hearing was better. My left ear which had been congested for years, and continually *popped* as I spoke, had cleared. It took me a whole month for my bowels to adjust to the increase in raw food. I have never been constipated since! I had so much more energy. My skin was also clearer than it had ever been. After initially losing a couple of pounds, my weight stabilised as it adjusted to the new dietary intake. This was all still whilst I was unaware of the benefits of nose breathing. Nose breathing would have naturally occurred more of the time without the extra mucus.

Five a Day is Not Enough

A more recent ten-year review[132] of medical research demonstrated that there is an inverse correlation between all epithelial cancers and fruit and vegetable intake. This means the more you have, the less likely you will get cancer whether the food is raw or cooked. It also showed there was a reduced incidence of breast cancer and upper gastrointestinal cancer when there is a higher percentage of raw food in the diet.[133]

When it comes to eating fruit and veg the five a day is not nearly enough. Yet it is surprising when I ask patients if they have a healthy diet, many answer, "Yes." And when I ask if they have their five a day, they often say, "Not every day." In one large study done in Australia (involving over 150,000 adults over the age of 45) with a follow-up six years later, showed that fruit and vegetable intake, both raw and cooked, significantly reduced mortality from all causes of disease, with the largest risk reduction seen in the people who had seven or more servings of fruit and vegetables per day.[134]

Many Nature Cure practitioners would suggest that for every decade of unclean living one year of clean living is required. Raw food is suggested to enhance the detoxification process and enhance our natural function. If you have an inflammatory condition in your system, raw foods can be incredibly cooling and don't produce as much mucus as the digestive leucocytosis is not occurring. It gives your immune system a rest. Cooking food can also create toxins within the food. It denatures vitamins and proteins, destroys vital enzymes needed for digestion and cellular function and increases the speed at which sugars are released from your food, as the cell membranes are more broken down.[135]

If you are not used to eating much raw food, I would suggest having two raw food meals per day is a good way to keep inflammation at bay. Once your body has become used to having two raw food meals per day over a couple of months, you could try having a couple of raw food days a week or a week every month of raw food, to help elimination. Finding out what works best for you is key. Eating every meal raw can cause some people to feel too cold. The food should never be eaten cold from the fridge, but warmed to 37 degrees around body temperature, to maintain enzymes and vitamins and make it more comfortable on our digestive system. Warm brown rice can be mixed with raw salad.

Feasting and Fasting

The practice of fasting has been around for millennia. Many religious groups adopted it for its health benefits. Naturopaths have been using it as a support to the healing process for centuries, once a healthier diet has been embraced. Recently science has been able to demonstrate how fasting benefits your health. Calorie restriction to around 1800kcal, combined with adequate nutrient intake, has been known for many years to increase health and longevity.[136,137]

There are correlations between raised Insulin Growth Factor 1 (IGF 1) and chronic health conditions and increased cellular replication.[138] Both fasting and a low-protein diet have been shown to lower IGF1 levels.[139] During fasting, IGF1 levels drop and cell replication slows down,[140] which gives the DNA a chance to repair itself before being passed on to the next cell generation. Long-term calorie restriction with high protein intake was not shown to lower IGF1 levels in human studies. However, low IGF1 levels may not be simply due to calorie restriction alone. In a group of long-term raw food vegans, lower IGF1 levels were demonstrated.[141] It is not just calorie restriction but the quality and type of food which will influence health.

Alternate Day Fasting

One significant study involved alternate day fasting with overweight adults with asthma. Calories were restricted on alternate days with impressive results after only two weeks. Peak expiratory flow (PEF)—the force of the out-breath—significantly increased. This has been shown to increase in some studies with Buteyko exercises,[142] but not in others.[143] Combining the breathing techniques with healthy eating is a great way to optimise your health. Alternate day fasting also reduced serum cholesterol and triglycerides—the blood fats, and markers of inflammation and oxidative stress in the body were considerably reduced. On the fast day women had 320 calories and men had 380. The following day the subjects ate their normal diet. Subjects lost around 8% of their body weight during the 8 weeks of the experiment. [144] PEF improved within the first 3-4 weeks when weight loss was only 4%. It was felt that the main improvement came from the anti-inflammatory response from the alternate day calorie restriction diet reducing airway hyper-responsiveness.

Along with reducing or eliminating the inflammatory ten foods, I would also recommend having alternate raw food days which will naturally limit the calorie intake. You could also have a vegetable juice day followed by normal food day. The healthier your foods are on the feed day, the better the improvement is likely to be.

Jamie was only fourteen months old when he came for treatment and had been put on inhalers for a few months due to breathing difficulties. His breathing symptoms had worsened with a head and chest cold. I suggested that he had a couple of weeks on raw food to help improve the breathing. Whilst laying on his front we also did some percussion on the back of his chest with cupped hands which helped to start moving the mucus and drain his lungs.

His mother was able to continue this and also continued doing some steam breathing with him in the bathroom. He made a rapid recovery on raw food after only three days. He went back to nursery, and after having a vegetable crumble, became rapidly worse. Again, improvement was made by removing wheat and dairy and increasing raw food intake. After a few days, he was able to come off his regular inhaler with the doctor's blessing, breathing normally once again.

The Right Time to Eat

Nature Cure and Naturopathy proposes that our body works in three distinct cycles which apply to our circadian rhythms.

- The digestive phase 12noon-8pm
- The assimilation phase 8pm-4am
- The elimination phase 4am-12 noon

It makes sense to help your body prioritise its functions as if you try to do more than one thing at a time it becomes inefficient. On waking your body has been working much harder during the night renewing and repairing tissues, which leads to increased elimination. This is why on waking many people have a more coated tongue, mucus congestion and the need to eliminate. If you break this fast immediately, it switches your body into digesting which takes the body's attention away from the eliminatory phase. By having a later breakfast or a light fruit or green smoothie breakfast, we can extend that eliminatory healing phase for longer.

Recent research has supported Nature Cure's age-old stance demonstrating that regulating when you eat and not just how much you eat can have significant effects on your health. It has been recommended that for the best health you should avoid eating for at least a sixteen-hour window each day.[145] If health improvement is your aim, some also suggest only eating within a 3-12 hour window each day.[146] The modern way of eating three meals per day plus snacks is not in line with our evolutionary development. We have been used to going without food during periods of scarcity. Modern convenience eating is a very recent occurrence and our escalating ill health is likely directly linked with overindulgence. In fact, we only really need to have two main meals per day.

Some Important Points to Remember

A true fast is a water-only fast. Never fast for more than three to four days on water only unless you are in a clinical setting. Fasting for more than three to four days if you take medication can make the medication more toxic to your system. Instead of fasting, you modify your diet to include more raw food, with cooked sweet potato and brown rice, and if your weight allows it, incorporate alternate day reduced feeding. Most people have three to four days of food in their intestines. Any fast longer than three to four days must *always* be supervised by an experienced practitioner, as breaking a fast should also be done at the correct time and with great care. You are not always in the best position to judge when you should break a fast. If you go longer, it could become seriously threatening to your health. Never overindulge after a fast or eat really heavy foods such as meat or grains. Your stomach will not appreciate the insult of a large meal straight after fasting. Keep it to fruit or vegetables.

If you have had a healthier diet for some time prior to fasting, you are less likely to have a severe reaction during a fast. There are many health conditions where chronic health doesn't afford enough vital reserve to enable fasting, such as in chronic fatigue. If your weight is already low, then fasting is inadvisable. It would be better to have a juice fast or a mono-diet during acute illness. Please consult a qualified health practitioner, experienced in giving guidance on fasting if you have a medical condition or health concern. For some people, even raw food can be difficult to digest. Having the right bacteria will help this, but some may fare better with cooked food, with a raw side dish or additional juices.

If you eat an entirely raw food, vegan diet, then over time the body can become deficient in vitamin B12. We have around 2-3 years of B12 reserves in the liver. B12 is essential for the myelin sheath that protects your nerves and also for the health of your red blood cells carrying oxygen around your body. Staying on a vegan diet long-term can be detrimental to the nerve and brain health. Probiotic bacteria in the gut can potentially help produce vitamin B12. However, I would never recommend relying on this alone. Long-term leaky gut also diminishes B12 absorption. It is contained in meat, fish, eggs and dairy produce, so unless you decide to eat some raw dairy, eggs or a couple of servings of raw fish each week, with your raw food diet I would recommend vitamin B12 supplementation is essential if you wish to be vegan.

When Should You Fast?

Fasting is indicated if you have lost your appetite when you have a chronic or acute illness and can also be used for psychospiritual reasons and even to break a habit. If you don't want to fast on a weekly basis then having two raw food days per week is an excellent way to cleanse your system. Regular fasting for children is not recommended, only if they have an acute crisis and have lost their appetite. Children generally respond well to a raw food approach for a few days after illness, once their appetite has returned. Adults require a more cleansing diet, whereas children are building their bodies and growing and need a slightly higher amount of protein in their diet for healthy growth.

For women, once menopause has been reached, the monthly elimination no longer occurs. In place of this, it would be advisable to still have a week each month where you actively have a cleansing approach to your eating, with either some fasting or raw food days. During menstruation is also a good time to support your elimination as the body is in a greater elimination mode at this time anyway.

However, I would suggest if you are serious about improving your health, have two raw food days per week and then in the following five days have two raw food meals per day, including breakfast and lunch, with some raw and cooked food for your evening meal. This is a great way to rebalance your body and improve your health. This will enable a better cleanse than eating 500 calories of more congesting cooked food. You can have an improved sense of fullness when munching through a plate of raw vegetables. The chewing action gives a greater feeling of satisfaction than when we eat soft cooked food.

If you have improved your health by eating a large amount of fresh, raw produce for a number of months—as long as you are not taking any medication—a water fast for 3-4 days with bed rest can be amazingly transformative if you are unwell. It is incredibly cleansing.

Tess came to the clinic experiencing severe asthmatic symptoms, upper back pain and blocked nose and she needed to use her inhaler on a daily basis. Asthma attacks were occurring frequently, whenever she smelt people's perfume or was exposed to dust and mould. After five days on a water fast, under supervision, followed by two days on a mono-diet, she has not needed to use her inhaler since. Three times a day, she did steam breathing to ease her lungs and nose congestion. She also used three simple Bowen technique moves to release her diaphragm. Her nose and lungs are no longer as reactive to the chemical smells, mould or dust in her environment and her back pain has cleared. As long as she eats healthily, her health remains.

As digestion expends large amounts of energy, fasting enables this energy to be diverted towards healing. Our system breaks down and eliminates cellular waste products before it metabolises the healthy tissue. Our body is intelligent—if it is treated with intelligence. And sometimes rest and an intelligent leaving alone is what is required.

Juice Fasts

If you are not ready for a water fast, juice fasts can be incredibly healing too and don't necessitate bed rest to avoid adrenal exhaustion. Never juice fast on fruit juices or shop bought juices as this will provide too much fruit sugar and they will not have the same nutritional value if they have been bottled.

Vegetable juicing helps to provide lots of micronutrients to the tissues of the body in an easily absorbable form in a large concentration. It is the healthy way to supplement your diet with minerals and vitamins that are alive. If the digestive system has become impaired from stress and eating congesting foods, having a juice fast can be a great way to cleanse the system and improve your health. Using a juice extractor, it is preferable to juice predominantly vegetables, rather than fruits so that we don't overconsume fruit sugars. Organic vegetables are ideal so that you are not taking in pesticides and fertiliser traces with your juice.

Mono-Diets

If you can't manage a juice fast, then a mono-diet is the next best thing to help with additional cleansing. If you are heavily congested with mucus but don't have a fever and don't have the ability to stop work and rest, you could eat watermelon only for 2-3 days. This helps to cleanse the whole system and is highly anti-inflammatory. If you don't like watermelon, then try cantaloupe melons instead. Watermelon is very cleansing for the kidneys. Asparagus also has the ability to kidney cleanse, which is why it can give an odour to our urine. When the urine no longer smells, then the waste has been eliminated. Having a mono-diet for a couple of days with a food that is simple to break down, enables the body to put most of its energy into healing and eliminating rather than breaking down heavy protein or carbohydrate meals.

A diet of just apples can also help to break down any stones in the liver. If the liver is eliminating more effectively, then the whole of our body becomes healthier. As non-organic foods can have high pesticide residues, please buy organic apples.

Rest

If you are fasting on water only you also need bed rest as the body will become overly stressed if you try to be active when not eating. Give yourself time to heal and relax and allow the process. Overstimulation from your surroundings is an extra strain on your nerves. Have some quiet time. This will enable you to rediscover your inner strength. Giving yourself time to stop and have a holiday without any pressure to do anything is sometimes exactly what is needed for our system to recharge.

It is better to eat well consistently than swing between extremes of overindulgence and fasting. If issues around food are related to emotional tension, then finding a practitioner to work with is helpful. Food can often be used too much for reward and punishment. If this applies to you, it may be more important to start with letting go of controlling your emotions with food first. Do the emotional work before addressing dietary intake. Then your choices towards food will be healthier and more in balance than they would have been with unresolved emotional issues in charge. The rewards felt in the moment of indulgence, often don't outweigh the consequences felt afterwards. Whatever you choose—let go of guilt. If you can't let it go completely with your food choice, then make a guilt-free choice. What are you punishing yourself for? Be kind and gentle with yourself.

When you feel under the weather, this is the time to really focus on making the most health-supporting choices. It is at this time that the body needs the most loving care and support. After all, if you want to have loads of energy for the many exciting opportunities in your life, you need to be able to give yourself the care and attention you need, when your body asks for it. It's just like stoking a fire. To get it roaring you need to put the best wood on it.

Finding a Balance

Living on a raw food diet and having a social life can be challenging. My friends and family were all very accommodating to my year on raw food, but in the end, I felt it was unfair to expect them to make special meals for me. At the end of the year on raw food, I continued having two raw food meals a day and went back to eating cooked food on an evening with occasional treats. I wondered whether the allergic response to animals would return. It did, but only when I overate, had cooked food or processed party food when I was in a house with pets or felt anxious.

I still give myself days on raw food to help support my body's natural cleansing process. It is so much more constructive to give yourself living, vital foods rather than suppress your natural reactions with drugs. I thought I had a really healthy diet before I had my year of around 80% raw food. It wasn't until I did this that I realised how much improvement in your health you can gain through a high raw food lifestyle. Just because you have to do it continually doesn't mean it is not a cure. You have to keep yourself clean on a regular basis by washing. You wouldn't wash yourself once and then decide that was the cure for keeping clean.

I was still eager to understand more about breathing health. I wanted to find a lasting way of reducing the stress and pressures on my system so that food didn't become the obsessive focus of my health. I knew I needed to stoke the fire, but once the fire was roaring, I wanted to keep it roaring. I did at least feel one step closer to resolving my health problems; land was in sight. There were two more important pieces of the jigsaw to find before I could truly breathe with ease. Whilst studying naturopathy I also undertook a postgraduate diploma in clinical hypnotherapy. The tools I learnt studying the subconscious and how to affect it would enable the healing to go deeper.

STEPS TO MASTERY—Week Three—Include Essential Vitamins

Include some foods containing B12 in your diet each week—either three eggs or up to 2-3 portions of wild salmon each week. Raw Nori (sushi seaweed) has been shown to contain viable B12.[147] However, dried Nori contains only B12 that is inactive in the body and in vegan children, processed Nori can deplete vitamin B12.[148] Shitake mushrooms also contain B12,[149] but a large volume is required. On a vegan diet, B12 supplementation is the only long-term solution. A methylcobalamin spray may be the best absorbed, but it is best to obtain your nutrients from natural foods. Some people find they have a histamine reaction to B12 supplementation. If goats' milk is tolerated, locating a source of organic, raw goats' milk would be ideal. Use this to make yoghurt or kefir.

PART FOUR—
THE MIND

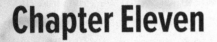

Chapter Eleven

Waking from the Trance

You use hypnosis not as a cure but as a means of establishing

a favourable climate in which to learn.

Milton H. Erickson

What is Hypnosis?

Hypnotherapy can be very helpful in supporting a conscious desire to achieve a particular goal or change our behaviours and habits. This may be, for example, to stop eating chocolate, and increase our natural desire to eat more healthily without battling our subconscious programmes. It is one of the most powerful ways of influencing your mind and thought processes, which in turn affect your behaviour and emotions. It gives you a feeling of focused attention with reduced peripheral awareness and increased suggestibility. Hypnotherapy is the use of hypnosis to transform a behaviour affecting a condition or a concern.

Hypnosis brings about mixed reactions from people. The word *hypnos* from Greek literally means *sleep*. A state of hypnosis is something we have all experienced. It is the state we enter when we have just driven down a section of road that is familiar to us, and we can't remember doing it. Most often this is because our mind is dissociated or split from the task at hand. This commonly happens during repetitive actions that have become habitual and is a natural state that we enter several times during the day. Hypnosis is an incredibly important part of our overall health and well-being as it safeguards our mind from being overwhelmed with information. It is a way in which our mind can process the vast amount of data it receives from our surroundings to enable normal, healthy functioning.

If you have ever walked down the street, thinking about what you did yesterday or what you are going to do later on in the day, you are in a state of hypnosis. Think about where your attention is whilst thinking about your past experience or future plans. If someone were to clap their hands, you would instantly come back to the present moment. Where does your consciousness go whilst you are focusing on something other than the present? As your energy follows your thoughts, part of your energy and attention is in the past memory or future event. This can be extremely helpful in resolving past issues or giving greater clarity to our forward progression, especially if we do this consciously. Imagining yourself on a beach, with the sea lapping against the shore, is also taking you into a natural state of hypnosis.

Hypnosis and Television

If you have ever been concerned about hypnosis, then I would suggest turning off your television. Hypnosis can be induced by concentrating on a point of focus. The old example of a swinging pendulum provides just that. Repetitive movement which catches our attention can induce a trance. Whilst we are watching television we have a point of concentrated attention, and our awareness is split from our body and focused on the screen.

This dissociated state of awareness, where our attention is split, is a state of hypnosis. In this dissociated state we often become less aware of our surroundings and become more suggestible, so if you are watching a traumatic scene, part of your consciousness will be experiencing it as though it is happening to you. You only have to see children transfixed on a television programme and how they act out the characters to realise how suggestible we are as young children and how they become hypnotised by a programme. This applies to adults as well. Otherwise, the advertising industry wouldn't exist. Watching adverts is a form of mind programming, and much of the language used in advertising is based on the understanding of implanting suggestions into your mind by associating the product with an implied emotional benefit. Suggestions are more likely to be accepted when there is a strong emotional association.

If we are watching without being consciously aware of what is being said, or questioning what we are told these suggestions can easily programme the population and change our habits. When we are consciously aware of our environment, it is quite incredible to realise how many suggestions there are around us that could be absorbed from our surroundings if we weren't consciously filtering them. The same applies to everyday life. As we are growing up, we are receiving programming about social conventions and acceptable behaviours even before we learn to talk.

Waking Up

Many people might think about hypnosis as putting someone *to sleep*. I look at it more as a way of waking you up from your old subconscious programming, so that you can be more awake and present in the moment. Rather than reacting from old programmes that might have occurred in your early years or whilst you were more unconscious, which can control your emotional reactions, you can find greater freedom to choose how you respond, rather than react.

It is important to understand that during clinical hypnotherapy it is always the intention that your subconscious will only accept positive, beneficial suggestions. Stage hypnosis is vastly different from clinical hypnotherapy. Stage hypnosis is designed to entertain and can demonstrate the power of the mind and how we can buy into a personality we experience as being *real*. Hypnosis can simply remove our inhibitions so that we feel freer to follow a new suggestion or internal programme. When we let go of our old programming, it is always important to replace it with something more positive and empowering. This could be as simple as replacing fear with happiness.

Turning the TV off and not watching the news, which can hold us in a state of fear, has been the best thing I could do to improve my mood and level of happiness. It doesn't serve anyone to watch people's suffering without taking action. Being unhappy about something doesn't help you or your family's happiness levels or the situation. We have to look at areas in our life that we can influence. If your circle of concern is larger than your circle of influence, you will feel stress. You either have to enlarge your sphere of influence or reduce your area of concern to reduce the gap and the tension associated with it. Learning to trust and believe in others and imagining them achieving their best is more empowering for them than worry for them.

When you are internally happy and content, you are more likely to make choices that are going to bring more of the same. The more people there are in the world who are living from a place of joy and happiness and able to give more joy to others by living consciously, the better the world will be. It is important to realise that your own positive thoughts also have the power to influence your behaviour. If you can choose your thoughts consciously, then you stand a better chance of staying connected to your joy and keeping your mind and body healthy. Why isn't it as simple as this? Why does positive thinking sometimes take such effort?

Repeated emotions can be due to old subconscious programmes that have developed from our early childhood experiences, which may maintain our present-day experiences. For example, a feeling of not being enough, or a fear of failure, can put enormous emotional pressure on you to perform. Imagine what it would feel like to release these fears of not being enough. Instead breathe in the feeling of being enough, knowing that whatever the outcome, you have done your best. When you discover what you believe in order to feel the way you feel, you have a choice to let go of the belief, to understand who you really are when you are free from that internal programme. As we mentioned before, the more naturally we allow the breath to flow, the easier the emotion will release. Slowing the breathing also helps to slow the mind.

Clearing Your Blocks

Sometimes people feel blocked from moving forwards with their health. For example, you may not give yourself time to do your breathing practice, or you might not fully commit to the healthy lifestyle changes that you know would make a difference. When you notice these contradictions inside you, you will be identifying that there is probably some subconscious belief that needs to change in order for you to value yourself enough to make that personal commitment. Sometimes the secondary gains we receive from being unwell are a factor in stopping us from moving forwards. At other times it might be that you give so much to others and don't give to yourself because you fear that might be selfish. You are worthy of your own time and commitment. It is the unconscious self-beliefs that have been keeping us in a trance that we need to wake up from. There may have been a part of you as a child that experienced love, care, affection and attention when you were ill. Sometimes we maintain a condition because our subconscious has learnt we can receive love and attention by being ill; the secondary gains mentioned earlier. It may be that you work hard to avoid feeling something.

People who overwork often find that they have a cold or illness when they have a holiday. The overwork could be driven by a need for success to gain love or approval, or the need to prove they are good enough, or a fear of lack. When we give ourselves permission to let go, the body will heal from the emotional tension often through a physiological release of extra waste. Every emotion has a corresponding chemistry and the more uncomfortable the emotion, the more acidic it is in our system. If you can identify what deep-seated fears are running the show for you, during hypnosis you can go beyond the fears and really connect to your true heart and find a new way of approaching your situation.

If you are not giving yourself the necessary love, care and attention that we often crave externally then illness is more likely to maintain. Focus on providing the needs for this part of you in a more wholesome way in order to let go of the need for the condition. This may involve re-parenting yourself—presenting yourself with the love and care you always wanted.

One person I met developed an inner dialogue with herself as though she were speaking lovingly to her daughter. Like many of us, we often speak more harshly to ourselves than to our loved ones. Speaking lovingly to yourself can enable all parts of you to be aligned with your vision.

You may resist lifestyle changes because of addiction to certain foods. These foods may be a substitute for lack of fulfilment in some area of your life. This is another area that may need some loving care and attention in order to resolve. Hypnosis can be a great way of being able to break through these addictions and find the love and connection within yourself that a part of you might be looking for externally.

Find Strength in Your Vulnerability

One of the stumbling blocks I discovered on my healing journey was that I recognised I was trying to *get rid* of the asthma as I fought the reactions and didn't want it to be there. If the asthma represented suppressed sadness, this is like trying to get rid of a part of you that forms an integrated whole. Imagine how a young child would feel if it was abandoned. Attempting to run away from an aspect of ourselves is futile. From an emotional perspective, an illness can be an expression of suppressed emotional vulnerability. Trying to rid yourself of your vulnerability is like trying to make yourself impervious to life. If the lungs are associated with the emotion of grief, and we resist feeling this emotion, the tension created by trying to stop feeling something will create irritation. You may also find that through the death of a loved one, love and sadness has become linked. Resisting the sadness blocks the connection to love. It is not a case of detaching them, but enabling the feeling of love to be greater than the feeling of sadness, so that you can hold all of the emotions without resistance, but with love, joy and harmony being the greater of these.

The other aspect to bear in mind is that you may be absorbing or breathing in too much from the world around you, trying to hold on to everything and forgetting to breathe out and let go. In this instance it is not the illness we are trying to destroy, it is redressing our emotional balance of taking in and letting go and allowing yourself to feel without judgement. In welcoming your vulnerability, you can access greater feelings of love and discover your true strength of heart.

Studies have shown a link between what you think and feel and how your body reacts. For example, in one study they hypnotised people to either feel sad, happy or angry. With each emotional state they then had a prick test with histamine; the inflammatory-causing chemical. When the people were hypnotised to be happy or angry, they reacted more slowly to the prick test than when they were sad.[150] In preschool children aged two to five years old, visual imagery and hypnosis significantly improved symptom severity of asthma but didn't decrease the frequency of attacks or alter lung function.[151] Getting your mind on board will, at the very least, help you to relax into tension rather than tense up against it. Unite this with your breathing retraining and you will start to transform your reality. It might be that it doesn't directly cure asthma, but if the asthma is brought about through underlying emotional tensions or even breathing higher in the chest because of bloating in the abdomen, then it could be used to support health improvements, which in turn will improve breathing.

Hypnotherapy and IBS

Hypnotherapy for IBS can be enormously helpful in addressing the underlying emotional component of IBS both in the short and long-term.[152] Research reported by the British Medical Journal showed a 71% improvement in IBS symptoms in the short term with 81% of those maintaining their improvement over the following five years. Of the remaining 19%, who had initially improved, there was only a slight deterioration experienced, with an overall improvement which had maintained. By having a short course of hypnotherapy for IBS, you could also improve your ability to breathe into your abdomen easily.

STEPS TO MASTERY—Week Four—Body Scan with Breathing

Self-hypnosis is easier than you might think. Go through a full-body relaxation during your breathing exercises, so you scan your body from head to toe, progressively relaxing yourself all the way through to achieve relaxation in body and mind. As you relax your body, you will relax your mind.

You can also hypnotise yourself by counting down from ten to one with each out-breath, becoming ten percent more relaxed with each number between ten and one. So that when you reach one, you will be fully relaxed. From here you can access your subconscious more easily. You can repeat your affirmations or mental rehearsal during your relaxation at least three times. You can bring yourself back to the room and back to full waking consciousness by counting yourself back up to ten as you breathe in on each number.

If you suffer from IBS related to emotional tension, consider having a course of hypnotherapy to resolve the IBS. When you reduce the amount of bloating you experience you will be able to breathe more easily using your diaphragm.

Remember, when you register this copy of your book you will be able to access lots of guided meditations and other resources linked to each section.

Chapter Twelve

Transforming Your Conditioning

Feelings come and go like clouds in a windy sky.

Conscious breathing is my anchor.

Thich Nhat Hanh

The Subconscious and Conscious Mind

Many people liken the mind to an iceberg; one third of the iceberg is visible above the water with two thirds hidden beneath the water. It is like this with the conscious and subconscious mind. The conscious mind being the part above the surface; the thoughts we are aware of. The vast majority of your subconscious mind is hidden from awareness; the part below the surface. Another way of thinking about this is to see the brain as the conscious part of your mind and the body, full of sensations, representing the subconscious mind. Learning to relax the tightening in the body can help to keep you in a place of ease.

Whether you are more in conscious or unconscious brain mode can largely be determined by your brainwaves. There are several different brainwaves states. They can be measured using electroencephalography or EEG sensors on the head.

Delta Brainwaves[153] 0.5-3 Hz

Delta brainwaves are the slowest, which usually occur in deep and dreamless sleep.

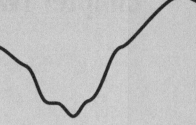

Theta Brainwaves[154] 3-8 Hz

Theta brainwaves occur during the dreaming stage of sleep, in deep meditative states and during hypnosis. They allow the mind to be highly suggestible.

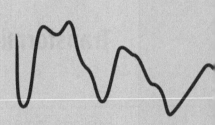

Alpha Brainwaves[155] 8-12 Hz

Alpha waves occur during daydreaming or whilst in creative imagination.

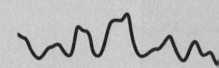

Beta Brainwaves[156] 12-38 Hz

Beta brainwaves occur during focused attention, especially whilst learning or in active thinking mode and are faster brainwaves.

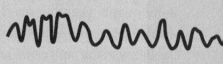

Gamma Brainwaves[157] 38-42+ Hz

There are also gamma brainwaves which occur in adults with heightened states of consciousness, for example when experiencing universal love.

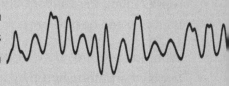

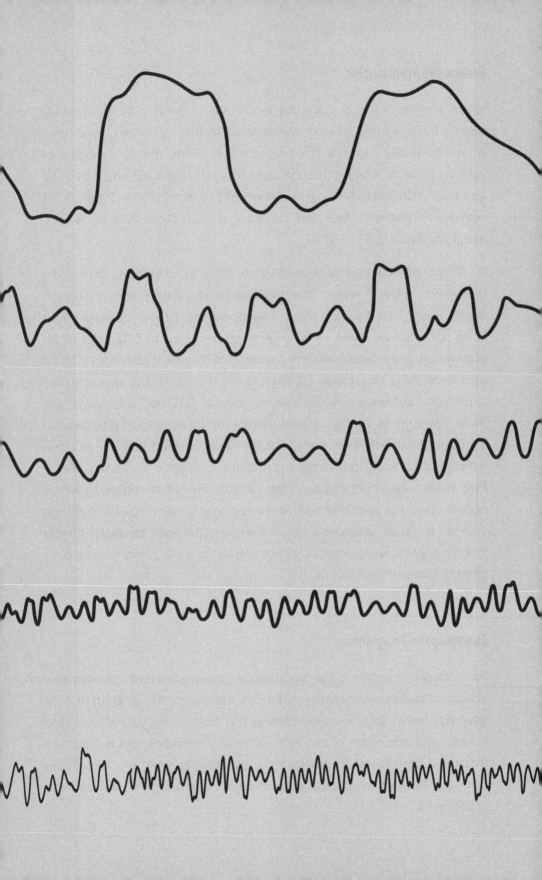

Brainwave Frequencies

When you are born, you are predominantly in delta state even whilst awake. Between the ages of five months to four years old, your brain waves gradually increase from around 3Hz in the first few months of your life in delta, moving through theta towards alpha, around 6-9Hz, by age four.[158] Children develop systematically towards higher frequencies with age.[159] Between four and six years old you move further into the alpha spectrum.

As states of hypnosis and meditation drop us into alpha and theta brainwave states,[160] where we become more highly suggestible, it would imply that through early childhood our brains operate more in an unconscious state of mind. Around the ages of 6-12 high alpha brainwaves are more consistent around 8-10Hz which coincides with us becoming more conscious. Through our teens from 13-19 years old we experience prolonged states of beta around 12-13Hz[161] where we are more *awake*. It is widely believed that even in adulthood only around 5% of our brain activity is conscious,[162] leaving around 95% of our brain activity determining our decisions, actions, emotions and behaviour.[163] EEG studies can demonstrate brain activity on decision-making which occurs up to ten seconds before we become conscious of it.[164] Giving yourself a pause to choose can make the difference between blindly following your subconscious programmes or being more awake to choose something different.

Changing the Programme

As much of our unconscious programming developed through what was absorbed during childhood experiences, the more you can learn to drop your brainwave state with meditation, the more likely you will be able to reprogramme some of the limiting beliefs, emotions and behaviours that have developed from that age. By slowing your breathing, you can actually start to quieten your mind and therefore slow down the brainwaves.

As adults, our perceptions of the future will in part be related to our past experiences.[165] Even the present is often perceived through the filters of our past. If we can be completely present to the moment without any preconceptions, we can begin to access new potential, and a new reality can unfold. If you have been banging on a closed door for a long time, maybe it is time to turn your attention to another door or window that might open for you.

If you have gone through strong emotional experiences in your early childhood, you may well have developed or absorbed beliefs and ideas about yourself and the world around you without question. These may have remained in your subconscious and become powerful drivers of your present-day experience. Some experiences will produce positive self-beliefs and others can create negative beliefs. These negative self-beliefs, which often run in the subconscious, can severely sabotage conscious positive thoughts. You can even choose new situations because they feel familiar because at some unconscious level you have experienced them before. This is absolutely fine if you have had positive experiences which you can replicate, but if you haven't, it can lead to repetitive cycles which you may wish to break free from. Slowing the mind to theta can enable you to access a more dreamlike state where you can be highly creative and come up with new solutions to your situation. You can be more receptive in a relaxed state. This is the state you enter into during hypnosis.

Hypnosis uses metaphors and images and sensory perceptions to gain access to the subconscious as you relax into deeper states of alpha and theta allowing you to experience heightened imagination and dreaming. Using hypnosis, you can safely access the memories where negative beliefs may have formed to enable you to release patterns of behaviour which were entranced within you. From there you can choose new empowering beliefs or states of being that will empower you. By waking yourself from your trance, you set yourself free to be more fully present and choose how you respond to life rather than react from your outdated subconscious programmes.

One of the ways in which you can wake yourself up from the trances of habitual activity is to become more conscious of how you do things. On waking, if you always get up and dressed in a particular order, try changing the order in which you do it, so you are more present. As you make small changes in your actions day to day, your mind will be able to create new pathways which can enable new future possibilities to arise.

Performance Anxiety

When there is a conflict between the conscious and subconscious mind, it often expresses as some form of tension in our body which activates the fight-or-flight nervous system. How conscious you are of these conflicts is a matter of how self-aware you are; a skill you can learn. Clearing out your limiting beliefs using hypnosis makes the act of mindfulness and present moment awareness much easier. Constantly battling old beliefs that challenge your positive attitude can be an uphill struggle.

If we are aiming to succeed in something whilst our subconscious has a fear of failure, this creates a tension between where you are and where you would like to be. Another example is having a desire to improve your health, but the subconscious programming contains a belief about lack of self-worth. In this way, it would be challenging to commit to positive changes until you learn to value yourself enough to make them long term.

If you have your subconscious working with you, feeling worthy, knowing that you can achieve what you put your mind to, you can enjoy the harmony of being present and calm, and your mind quiet and peaceful. Suggestions for new states of being can either be presented by a hypnotherapist, or you can imagine them yourself and breathe in what it feels like to have the new inner response during self-hypnosis. This can enable your elephant (your subconscious mind) and the rider (your conscious mind) to work together.

It wasn't until I came to re-evaluate where my biggest stress responses were arising from that I identified that I had been running almost my entire life from a fear of failure. This had started during my teenage years when I had put myself under massive pressure to achieve because I was looking for external validation. A perceived subconscious feeling of inferiority combined with a fear of failure can be a strong driving force which pushes us harder and harder to reach some almost unobtainable future reality that we strive for. Looking for external validation means putting your self-worth in the hands of others. When these fears and unconscious beliefs were challenged in me, it felt like a physical pain of being stabbed through the heart. If at times like this you can realise that it is an old story surfacing, which is probably based on a lie, and transform your old pain through self-compassion rather than self-pity you can become free of these stress-inducing patterns.

Having breathed and relaxed through the pain, having expanded it outwards, you can then breathe into your heart what it feels like to already be exactly where you need to be and have self-worth. Give yourself the inner validation and affirm that, *who you are in each and every moment is enough.* Being present to the truth of who you are, you may even receive words from your own heart to guide you forwards. Magic and miracles exist in this place. Often when you break through an old, painful pattern, you are able to see it for the illusion it really was. The fear can then no longer control you, and your heart can fill with love for you. When you are in this place, no external validation is required.

Living more consciously means being aware of what you are feeling in each moment and having a commitment to yourself to enable change to happen. Often change is more comfortable when we work with issues that feel manageable and can see our progress step by step. When we meet with a core issue, such as fear of failure or our core rage, or fear of losing our mind, and move through it to a place of peace, we can make significant steps forwards. It doesn't always happen in just one process. There is a continual cleaning of our internal self. There is an end to the process. You will find the more you clear, the more spacious and light you feel inside. The more you clear, the more present you become, the deeper the listening and the clearer the insights will be. You also create space inside of you so that you can listen more deeply to others, then you can be a support to others who may be struggling.

Hypnotherapy is therefore not about putting us to sleep. It helps you to wake up to your limiting beliefs and self-sabotage. It can help transform the fears or phobias which obscure your true self and enable you to become more conscious of the choices you make to awaken to your full potential.

To be intensely present in the moment requires a clear mind and a high level of awareness or mindfulness. As your breathing reacts to your stress response, finding ways of responding rather than reacting enables you to break free of your conditioned responses and awaken from the trance.

Changing Your Habits

Your subconscious—your body consciousness—may remember the pleasure associated with unhealthy food you have eaten, but you can easily learn to forget this and find healthier pleasures. Our brains are hardwired to find food that will carry us through times of drought and famine. Now there is an overabundance of food available, life-enhancing choices need to be made. With hypnosis, you can release the struggle between the conscious mind and the subconscious desire which might previously have caused tension and increased your stress levels. It is so much easier to let go of this struggle and make healthy choices that you can feel proud of. I call food that contains no real health benefit—as it is devoid of essential vitamins and mineral—*foodless* food, as it takes more from your body than it provides. If you haven't had *foodless* food for a few weeks, it is easy to forget any cravings because the addictive substances have left your body.

It is possible during hypnosis to clear your desire for sweet foods or whatever your particular weakness may be. Just as you may look at your least favourite food and have no desire for it, with hypnosis you can feel the same about foods you may have previously craved. I am certain that by clearing the habitual, addictive programming of emotional eating through hypnotherapy it makes it so much easier for me to stay on track with a healthy lifestyle. It takes away those subconscious drives to eat unhealthy food. I could simply look at a cake and choose not to have it, without any feeling of lack, because my subconscious and conscious minds were working in cooperation with each other. I can choose health; so can you.

Whilst in an open, receptive, relaxed state you can bring the subconscious on board with your lifestyle changes, by finding hundreds of alternative behaviours that bring the same or even greater benefits than chocolate or salty, savoury snacks. After all, who said a treat has to be food. Sugar and love have been associated many times with each other throughout childhood, but external sweetness is not the same as having internal sweetness or kindness for yourself. Isn't it better to aspire to something other than food as a reward for your efforts at work or with the family? Surely experiences are the things which really stay with us? You can achieve your goals more easily, without the internal battle of willpower. When you give your mind and body the *thought* along with the associated *feeling* that your choices are positive empowering ones, the battle ceases.

You can also choose healthier food options for your treats. For example, instead of chocolate, I choose delicious Medjool dates. Instead of crisps, I enjoy a few olives or some kale chips. You can also give the suggestion to the subconscious that man-made sugary foods are sickly sweet. Refined sugars are far too sickly sweet for the natural taste buds that have learnt to savour the sweetness of a fresh, crisp apple or even notice how sweet carrots are. Rewards could be taking a walk in the sunshine, or taking time to read a book or have a bubble bath or massage. Spend some time with your friends playing badminton, have some time in the garden or relax with a good film. You can take your relaxation response into your daily life and become more mindful of living from that space.

Worry

Unconscious worry is possibly one of the greatest threats to health— possibly another thing to worry about! Overthinking things or living with an uncomfortable uncertainty places a huge strain on the body's systems. Having had times of deep relaxation during hypnosis, it can be easier to spot the contrast when worried thoughts start to surface outside of hypnosis or meditation. In fact, you may begin to notice how much of your time is spent worrying about things that are outside of your control.

Trying to stop yourself from worrying is futile because it involves the effort of thinking you have to do something to clear your mind. Catching the thoughts and smiling at your mind chatter is a light-hearted way of playing with the thoughts rather than using energy to fight the thoughts. Make friends with your mind. As we realise the game our mind is playing, smiling at these old stories and programmes enables you to let them go more easily, a little like throwing a stick into a stream. We can then allow the thought to pass or replace it with a more conscious, positive thought that enables you to relax and let go and trust or take the necessary action. Worry can be caused by having a large circle of concern, with only a small circle of influence inside that. You either have to increase your circle of influence to the size of your circle of concern or reduce the size of your circle of concern to reduce your stress levels.

Ultimately, to allow your life to flow it is important to let go of the illusion you have control over everything. This can bring fears to the surface, but the more controlled you are, the more tense you will be. As you relax the tension, imagine you can ask the controller in you for permission to let go. You can ask your higher self to flood you with a feeling of ease and release. For me the opposite of worry is trust.

If all else fails, remembering that you probably can't remember what you were worried about this time last year can help. If you are worried about someone else, it is far more empowering to envisage a positive outcome to their situation than worst-case scenarios.

Unconscious beliefs often underlie worries, and it is easy for beliefs to be unconscious because they are the basic assumptions and stories we tell ourselves about the way life is. Often our subconscious tries to protect us with the beliefs we have. If your mind comes up with worst-case scenarios, you may feel more prepared or guarded with the many different outcomes in your mind. However, it takes an enormous amount of energy. By staying relaxed and trusting life, we are likely to be more open-minded and creative. Should a challenge occur in our lives, we will be more open to finding a creative solution if we are relaxed than if we already feel burdened with countless other imaginary stories. Unless we question the validity of these stories, we may continue to sabotage our health and well-being for no good reason.

If the awareness comes from your head chatter, it is likely to be a worry. If you suddenly get a bodily reaction, then a sense about something and it won't release, then be guided by your intuition and higher self. During meditation, you can dialogue with the part of you that is infinitely wise. This may help you see the bigger picture which we sometimes can't from our limited human perspective. I imagine handing my worries over to a power greater than me which intends the best possible outcome.

Whenever you catch yourself worrying, please don't berate yourself. This simply increases internal tension. Just catch yourself and smile at your mind chatter. Then reach for a new feeling and a more empowering belief or story about your life, and feel what it feels like to be living from this place. You can internally speak to your body every time you catch yourself worrying by saying, "Thank you and I choose trust." This can then become your new reality.

The False Floor

Having a stressful start in life can create an early set point within the nervous system. Coming into the world can be associated with fearing life, the unknown, or not being loved. When faced with not being loved or the unknown the body goes back to the early programmed response that is preverbal. Our reactivity is going to be on red alert. In order to access theta or delta brainwaves with your breathing meditation, you need to shift your set point to one of greater relaxation and trust. You may be one of those people who just can't sit still for any length of time and rest because when you do, the nervous tension arises.

If there was a great deal of tension at the start of your life, it might have left you feeling ungrounded. This could be described as a *false floor*. When a baby is held by a mother who feels anxious, they don't relax in their mother's arms. When placed on the floor, they don't trust the floor to hold them, and they don't trust life to support them. With the whole system on red alert, it can eventually become exhausting. If this is the case with you, then working on grounding and feeling connected to the earth beneath you is essential. Lying on your back and feeling the earth holding you and supporting you will help to find more connection and peace of mind. Sitting upright and feeling your feet on the floor whilst at the same time feeling unconditional love showering through an imaginary funnel in the top of your head and down through your body, is a great way to reconnect to trusting the flow of life within you.

Changing State

During a state of hypnosis, you can access different emotional states that you might not have consciously experienced before. Using your imagination, you can create new internal states or inner resources which you can then draw from. You can experience what it feels like to *be* love, what it feels like to feel safe and relaxed when alone, what it feels like to be heard and acknowledged, all of which may replace previous earlier experiences of the opposite feelings. This enables you to transform how your body functions so that you can stay calm and relaxed with triggers that previously would have caused a reaction.

One process that I find very beneficial is the *Control Room of the Mind*. You can imagine a house and enter the attic room which is the control room of your mind. It contains levers and dials that represent the controls for the many different internal processes going on inside your body. You could tweak the levers and dials to regulate your body responses. You can get as creative as you like. You could even choose to let go of control and set one of the dials to freedom from control. You may wish to do this with a practitioner so that you feel held, supported and guided through this process. When you have someone guide you, you can often go into a deeper state of relaxation, which can have a more profound and lasting effect.

Treasure Chest

With hypnosis, you can dive deeper into your ocean of awareness and find your treasure chest. Your treasure chest represents your internal sense of knowing that at the core of your being, your very essence is love. Not romantic love, but simply the pure energy of connection to *All That Is*. Rather than being tossed around on the surface with a shark circling your iceberg, you can drop beneath your fears, or sharks, and connect to a oneness deeper than the surface emotions and waves and rest in the stillness and truth underneath and find your treasure chest. When you open your chest, you can feel the radiance within.

Memory and Conditioning

If you have experienced a particular reaction repeatedly it is easy to assume that this is the way life is. We may have particular triggers that bring on a stress response. Every time I went to a friend's house, my breathing would become tight-chested because they had spaniels just like Goldie, the cocker spaniel that I would cuddle at my grandmother's house whilst she was terminally ill. My subconscious mind automatically linked this with the story of my younger experience. The smell of dogs was enough to trigger this response. I would immediately become aware of my breathing, it was no longer relaxed. I also noticed I wanted to switch to mouth breathing, but kept it slow with nose breathing.

During a breathing meditation workshop, I recognised the smell of dog was associated with the fear of death and dying that had got linked with Goldie as I would curl up with her in her basket whilst my grandmother was dying. As I breathed through these remaining fears triggered by smell, which is connected to our emotional brain, I was able to relax through them and come to a deeper sense of peace. I could now tell my subconscious it was just the smell of dog and it was safe to relax. After releasing the fear during meditation, I went round to my friend's house and ate a cooked meal without wheezing at all. I kept my solar plexus relaxed, as I had noticed it was tensing there when I felt anxious about a situation which caused me to breathe higher in my chest instead of into my abdomen. Keeping the nose breathing slow and steady and into your tummy enables you to breathe with ease.

Smell and memory are deeply linked in the limbic system which has links with the hypothalamus, which is at the top of the autonomic nervous system. This could activate a stressed breathing response, as smell triggers the old memory that is associated with the memory of the old stressful situation. This is the *Pavlov's dog* conditioning which can affect our internal physiology. This process happens without engaging the conscious mind. Pavlov's dog was an experiment in which they rang a bell

173

every time they brought food for the dog. Eventually, the dog would start salivating whenever they rang a bell. The association had been made between the ringing of the bell and the arrival of food. This is known as a conditioned response. It shows that your body's reactions can be conditioned by stimulus or a thought. It made me realise how much your memories and associated emotions can have an effect on your state of health. If you allow yourself the possibility of a new reality, you can begin to find cracks in the old story which allows room for change and takes away the fear that was controlling you in those situations. This can give you a renewed confidence in what is possible.

Our Contradictions

Start noticing any contradictions you hold. For example, you may want good health, but you may not love yourself enough to let go of the habits you know are harmful to you. You may want more energy but constantly keep yourself in a state of overwork or pressure with deadlines. You may wish to feel happier in your relationships but treat yourself poorly and harshly judge or criticise yourself for not being good enough. There are countless examples of how we may have these opposing thought processes, which cancel each other out and sabotage our potential to bring our dreams to reality. Finding the point at which this started and going back to the memory where the feeling of not being good enough started, and breathing in a new, more conscious understanding into that memory I have found to be profoundly transformative. It helps to align and integrate the past subconscious with the present consciousness.

It is simply time to catch the game you play so that you can let it go and create a new conscious reality. You are vastly more powerful than you have ever realised. In order to be in a state of ease, you must bring about an integration of these opposites. You may go to one extreme or the other, but in the end, welcoming the full spectrum of who you are, enables you to find a way back to your centre.

Creating an Empty Space for Something New

Your personality is developed very early on in your life. It can occur through learnt behaviour and is always looking for your basic needs to be met. You may perceive that your needs have to be met by your external reality, which puts you at the mercy of changing external circumstances. When you have a clear connection to an internal source of strength then, no matter what happens externally, you still know internally that you are safe and well. You have found an aspect of you that is deeper than your personality; your authentic individuality.

The personality always fears its demise and will often put up a bit of a fight to prevent its own ego death. This dying to the old ways is necessary to be able to move forwards into something new. When it comes to endings, struggling never makes it easier. Let go and fly.

Rapid Induction of Hypnosis

If you feel tension in your chest, it isn't a solution to have to get to your hypnotherapist to overcome an attack. However, with some preparation and learning how to induce self-hypnosis, you can do a lot to release tension from your body. You might find yourself in a situation where it isn't possible to sit down and go through a twenty-minute guided meditation to recentre. Luckily, there is a way to rapidly induce hypnosis and relaxation. There is an eye-roll reflex which is used in hypnosis and in the Buteyko Method which enables you to gain instant relaxation.

As long as you have no eye problems and are not wearing contact lenses, if it is safe to do so, you can start by closing your eyes and focusing on the point just between your eyebrows for a few seconds. Then keep your eyes closed and look up to the roof of your head for about 20-30 seconds. Using the relaxation, in the pause at the end of your out-breath, to enhance the relaxation feel your bottom sink into the chair or your feet connect with the ground. Then relax your eyes. You can use this to lengthen your control pause or simply to release tension from your chest. I imagine sending the tension up and out through the roof of my head.

I found this particularly helpful to reduce abdominal discomfort when I started eating a diet with more raw food in it. I lay partly propped up in bed, and with my eyes closed, I looked down into my abdomen as I breathed into it. Then I imagined scooping up the tension with my gaze and sending it up and out through the top of my head as I looked upwards and breathed out. Within a few breaths, the pain had gone. If you are able to do this, it can be incredibly relaxing, whether you are in pain or not. You can relax your mind to relax your body, or you can relax your body to relax the mind. The eye-roll scoop was one of the main steps in creating the Dynamic Breath Release.

STEPS TO MASTERY—Week Four—Eye-Roll

Listen to the Control Room of the Mind guided meditation and use the eye-roll during the meditation to help you to go deeper into relaxation. If you have any abdominal tension or discomfort, look down into it on the in-breath. On the out-breath scoop the tension up with your vision and send the discomfort up and out of your head. You can imagine or see what colour it is and send the colour out. Now breathe in a new healing colour in its place. Remember to soften and relax the centre of your chest in the pause at the end of your out-breath.

Caution: Do not do the eye-roll if you have an eye condition or are wearing contact lenses.

Chapter Thirteen

Mindful Awareness

You cannot solve a problem from the same consciousness

that created it.

You must learn to see the world anew.

Attributed to Albert Einstein

Thoughts Become Reality

If your thought process can make you ill, what thought processes would you need to choose in order to be well? When you catch yourself thinking a particular thought process that causes you tension and stress, in that moment you have the choice to be able to reach for a better feeling thought. Often the small choices you make every day build up to be the big choices that make the difference between health and dis-ease in the long run. These can be choices such as what food you eat, when you go to bed, if you choose to have a walk or even the thoughts you choose.

You are not at the mercy of your mind, you can be the observer of your mind. This is what mindfulness practice can teach you. You can grow from all the experiences you have and gain wisdom.

How Much Stress Builds Before You Notice It?

Sometimes people don't notice how they are stressed until it gets to the point of overwhelm or until after the stress has been resolved and the relief is felt. Stress in the mind reflects in the body, packaged up as physical tension or potentially creating symptoms of dis-ease—as your body chemistry responds to the stress and makes adaptive changes. Through meditation and relaxation exercises, you can relax and let go more fully. This is a great way to start practising living with greater presence and become more mindful of your reactions. If you can catch the thought as it arises, you can choose whether you engage with it or not. Mindfulness meditation also teaches us how to quieten the mind so that you can listen to what your body-mind is communicating with you.

The Power of Acceptance

We live in a world of duality. This means that without darkness there would be no light. One defines the other. Who you really are in your essence is beyond the dualities of good and bad, black and white. Having a direct experience of this will give you a full understanding of the truth of your existence. It is the ego that wants to cling to definitions of good or bad. Superego is the judge of the behaviour. Your superego arises when you start judging what others do or even what you are doing. Both can be just as limiting. Being the observer, without judgement, is the aim of mindful, meditative practice. If you find yourself experiencing a judgement of a situation, it will be interesting to notice where you tense in your body in relation to this thought. It is almost like the body defends itself against the hostility of the mind. You can release the tension by befriending your mind. Mindfulness practice involves scanning the body to release areas of tension whilst being the observer of your body and mind. I like to do it with playful curiosity. One definition of mindfulness presented at a mindfulness-based stress-reduction class was:

"Seeing what is happening in the mind, as it is happening

without judgement or preference."

The whole of life has a preference for one thing over another, it is built into our evolution, and therefore it is likely to be impossible to eradicate stress altogether. It is the long-term stress that chronically sits inside us that becomes the health issue. Stress arises in the mind when we start to believe that one way is better than another, or someone else's preference is better or worse than ours.

Rather than allowing thoughts, feelings and emotions to cause you to be swept away, becoming aware of your thoughts before they feed into emotions, without self-criticism or judging them, can be helpful in allowing you greater creativity to resolve them. This means that if you are suffering, by beginning to accept and reconnect with what you are feeling, rather than pushing away and making the pain or tension wrong you can begin to unite your mind and body once more. This creates wholeness or healing.

From a relaxed body, you can then begin to notice when areas tense with particular thoughts. If you notice a judgement or thought about what you are feeling, you can begin to discover what thoughts or beliefs may be maintaining your stress. For example, when my breathing is wheezy *I feel......(emotion)........which makes me think......(belief).........*(fill in the blanks). There is no right or wrong way to be feeling at any given time. Having observed this thought process, can you let it go with the breath?

What happens to you if you relax your whole body and then welcome *all* thoughts to surface? Anything? Nothing? Emptiness? Welcoming thoughts enables your mind to come to rest. Becoming comfortable with an internal emptiness or nothingness is often what the overwhelmed mind and body needs to rest. This creates a space for something new to emerge. During *Mind-Fullness* what essential quality would you like your being to be full of? Contentment? Peace? Love? Joy? You can choose.

Sometimes when you meditate, it can feel like more thoughts are happening. However, it could simply be that rather than a background hum of mental activity, you are able to pick out the individual thoughts as your mind slows. This is a little bit like having a fan whirling on the ceiling, and as it slows down, you can see the individual blades. Eventually, it will come to rest as you observe it, without having to do anything.

Focusing on the sensations and feelings in my body that were related to various thoughts passing through my mind, I was amazed to discover how interconnected they were. I had previously seen my thoughts and my physical sensations as separate. I now began to see how they were interconnected. This union of mind, body and emotion has been known to many for millennia and is described in India as yoga. Yoga meditation has been shown to reduce metabolic rate and oxygen consumption.[166] Another study in the 1980's showed that through transcendental meditation, oxygen consumption dropped by as much as 40% and breathing rate dropped by 50% during meditation.[167]

If you are choosing the stress that you are experiencing, then it is less stressful than someone in a situation they feel they haven't chosen, which puts them in more of a victim place. The truth is we all have the power to choose. All choices have consequences, which could turn into new opportunities, especially if you have felt like you are going round and round in circles. Try breaking the cycle by doing something different.

For me the opposite of judgement is acceptance. This doesn't mean rolling over in defeat, it simply means seeing the situation as it is and accepting how you are feeling right now. If the situation you find yourself in is unacceptable to you, then notice what you are thinking in order to feel that way. Thank your thoughts for protecting you. Notice where you are tensing in your body and soften and relax. As you bring your attention into the body, the thought often releases as the tension does and vice versa. This is one way of reconnecting your mind to your body. Breathe, let go and then choose a new thought or feeling. You are the observer of this process. You are not your thoughts. A short mindful process you could do if a thought has made you feel sad is to breathe into the emotion, in this case, sadness, then breathe out sadness. Breathe in sadness, then breathe out love. Then breathe in love and breathe out love. It is a simple process of acknowledging how you are feeling and choosing something different. More often we learn more from our failures than our successes. If you have a curiosity for what you can learn from each experience, you will be more open to life. Not having a preference means that you decide to accept what you are thinking and feeling in this moment and live in harmony with whatever arises. It is only your ego that gets caught up in desires for something different.

The Stress Response

Increased breathing rate will increase the stress response in the body as it shuts down circulation to the brain.

Brain scans have been used to demonstrate a significant reduction in blood flow to the brain after one minute of hyperventilation.[168] This reduction in blood flow could explain why you could experience brain fog or a reduction in memory and cognitive reasoning with a stress response and hyperventilation. Changes in brain blood flow have been backed up in functional MRI studies. It was shown that, "Changes in respiration associated with anxiety.... can produce local and global changes in cerebral blood flow that is unrelated to regional neuronal activation."[169] This means the circulation changes in the brain were not related to nerve activity but to breathing excessively in relation to the anxiety state. If the blood flow can change so quickly with stress, with the ability to relax and let go with the breath, blood flow could also be quickly and easily restored. With better breathing, the blood flow returns and restores our higher brain functions. Cerebral blood flow changes can occur rapidly with small changes in our oxygenation and carbon dioxide levels.[170]

Changes to blood flow in the brain could also trigger headaches. Migraines occur when there has been a constriction of blood flow, followed by a rapid dilation. If there has been emotional holding or tensing in an area of the body without us being aware of it, it will be in these places that we suffer the most when we breathe more rapidly with stress. Often migraines come about with digestive upset, and in my personal experience can coincide with mental indecision and striving for perfection and exhaustion.

James found that having suffered migraines for many years, which had increased in frequency to once a week, a lifestyle change was needed. He had weekly osteopathic treatment for one month, followed by fortnightly for another couple of months and then on a monthly basis for a year to adjust his neck and relieve upper back tension. He also cut out food that he was intolerant to, including dairy, yeast, sugar, wheat and eggs. He started having a fruit breakfast every day, a salad lunch and cut out alcohol, tea and coffee. His migraines have stopped and have remained at bay for the last three years. His days of taking paracetamol on a weekly basis have long gone, and he hasn't required any for the last three years. He maintains his health through healthy eating and regular meditation and exercise.

If you have a headache, imagine breathing in and out quietly and slowly from the centre of the pain, whilst welcoming the sensation and allowing it to dissipate outwards in the pause at the end of the out-breath. Similar to releasing the tension from the chest, this can be applied to areas of discomfort throughout the body. Don't fight the pain, the tension increases the experience. Make sure you are properly hydrated and whatever your decisions in life, choose them wholeheartedly.

Experimenting with Mindfulness and the Breath

I was fascinated to discover how much of a difference using mindfulness practice during meditation makes to your breathing rate and control pause. During my advanced Buteyko training, I set up an experiment with twenty-nine volunteers from people who had previously visited me at York Natural Health for osteopathic treatment. The participants were informed that they would measure and record the effects of mindfulness meditation on their breathing.

The number of breaths in one minute was recorded before and after a twenty-minute meditation, with a control pause measurement at the start and end of the meditation. Following a normal in-breath, the control pause is the length of time you can comfortably pause from the end of the out-breath to the next in-breath. This was measured by counting the beats of a metronome, set to sixty beats per minute, during their pause.

The control group included nine people who took their measurements before and after sitting quietly in a separate room for twenty minutes. The experimental group of twenty people took their two measurements and recorded them before and after a twenty-minute guided mindfulness body scan meditation, where they were instructed to focus on each area from their feet up to their head and relax each area in turn.

The average breathing rate reduced by 17% in the control group and by 28% in those in the guided mindfulness body scan group. Slower breathing indicates a greater level of relaxation. Although the length of the control pause was increased in both groups at the end of the session, the control group had an average increase of 20% in length of control pause, whilst the guided meditation group had an average increase of 42% in the length of their control pause. It would appear that there is great value in having someone audibly guide you through a process of relaxation. It can help the mind to relax more as someone holds the space for you to let go more deeply. Sitting in silence may work very well for experienced meditators, and although slowing down and taking time out to do nothing is helpful, those effects can be significantly enhanced by listening to guided mindfulness meditation. It may also indicate the power of a larger group meditation.

STEPS TO MASTERY—Week Four—Use the Body Scan and Breathe into Areas of Tension

Use the body scan during your breathing practice to enable your body to soften and relax. You can work from your feet upwards or your head down as you relax each part in turn. Listening to the guided meditation may help you to relax more.

If you notice any tension or discomfort in your body, try breathing into it and softening and expanding the area as you pause at the end of your out-breath. Welcome what you are feeling so you don't fight the tension. Having no preference for something means you can still choose healthy choices for yourself, it would be better described as a radical acceptance of *what is* or a surrender to a situation, when you are in a safe place. Just in this moment don't try and change what you are feeling.

PART FIVE—
THE BREATH

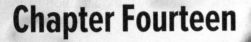

Chapter Fourteen

The Space to Breathe

We shall not cease from exploration,

and the end of all our exploring will be to arrive where we

started and know the place for the first time.

T. S Eliot

Revisiting Buteyko

Have you ever felt that if only you could take a deep enough breath, you would be fine? In that case, you need to retrain your breathing. I used to be quite familiar with this feeling; however hard I struggled my lungs seemed to act like a cage around me that prevented me taking a deep enough breath to feel free. It wasn't until many years of asthmatic episodes that I suddenly realised that in order to be free I had to surrender. I had experienced the surrender into the water as I had felt myself drowning in my meditation which had enabled my lungs to switch from an asthma attack to feeling as though my breath went on forever, but I had never managed to reproduce the experience until my breakthrough seven years later. It was my own modification of the Buteyko Method that enabled this to be possible.

I first came across an article about the Buteyko Method around the time I was finishing my degree in osteopathy around 2003. I had heard about the practice of holding the breath to help relieve asthma but when I tried it, without proper instruction, for the first time whilst wheezing it seemed to just make my breathing worse. I was holding for only a couple of seconds, but when I started breathing after the breath hold, I had an even greater wheeze and need for air and was gasping for breath.

It wasn't until eight years later that I revisited the work of Professor Buteyko to learn more. Bringing together what I had studied over the previous decade with my understanding of the Buteyko Method I experienced a life-changing discovery. I overcame an asthma attack in three minutes. In this synchronous moment, everything came together for me. I can't really say I overcame it, more I stopped fighting my body's reaction. I found a deep inner peace. Before explaining how you too can experience this breakthrough, first a bit of history.

Professor Konstantin Buteyko (1923-2003) was a Russian doctor who had observed that in chronic disease patients nearly always suffered from hyperventilation, also described as *overbreathing*. Their breathing rate was increased, occurring mainly in the upper chest and remained shallow or high volume. He found that by retraining their breathing and reducing the amount the patient breathed he could improve many different health conditions, not just asthma. As asthma is a breathing-related condition, it is an obvious focus for the retraining; however, it has benefitted people with other long-term health problems where there is chronic *hidden* hyperventilation syndrome. It is hidden because you may not always be aware that you are doing it.

Dysfunctional breathing can affect as many as one in ten people.[171] The Nijmegen Questionnaire[172] gives an indication of symptoms associated with chronic hidden hyperventilation. It is referred to as hidden because it isn't always obvious to the person that they are breathing so rapidly. Hyperventilation syndrome can cause symptoms such as difficulty breathing, chest tightness, chest pain, palpitations, blurred vision, dizzy spells, bloated feelings in the stomach, tingling fingers, stiff fingers or arms, feelings of tightness around the mouth, cold hands or feet, feeling tense or feelings of anxiety.[173] Functional heart problems have also responded well to breathing retraining.[174] In some cases, hyperventilation can be mistaken for epilepsy and complex partial seizures,[175] as there is often a hyperventilation component as part of the aura.[176] Buteyko himself retrained his breathing to lower his high blood pressure. Slow breathing has been demonstrated to be highly effective at lowering blood pressure or hypertension.[177,178,179] Fatigue symptoms have also been shown to be significantly related to hyperventilation in response to emotive triggers.[180]

Buteyko's Russian colleague Alexander (Sasha) Stalmatski brought this method to the UK in the 1980s. In 1998 the Buteyko Method was presented on a BBC Documentary. It has been recommended by the British Thoracic Society (BTS) as a "breathing practice which can help reduce the symptoms of asthma." [181] The Buteyko Method was found to reduce asthma symptoms and bronchodilator use in four separate clinical trials.[182,183,184,185] The Scottish Guidelines (SIGN) also recommend Buteyko in their *Breathing Exercises for Asthma*.[186] Buteyko has been approved by GINA, the Global Initiative for Asthma, as a breathing technique that has shown improvements in symptoms and is given an A rating for the level of evidence.[187]

Endings and New Beginnings

I had struggled with allergic asthma my whole life, and when many of my close family members had pets, it gave me even more incentive to try to overcome the problem. However, the harder I tried to breathe into my abdomen the worse my breathing became. Trying to *out-breathe* an asthma attack just caused further tension to build. I couldn't understand what I was doing wrong. I had learnt it was good to breathe deeply. After all, doesn't it mean we bring in more oxygen? That was my misconception until I started reading about the Buteyko Breathing Technique (BBT).

I knew that if I didn't eat cooked food or drink fruit juice whilst in the presence of animals my immune system could cope without producing an allergic, asthmatic response. Eating a high raw food diet enabled me to breathe with ease, but I knew that there must be another key to helping maintain my breathing in a normal healthy range, just as other people did. Even though I tried to relax with hypnosis, it helped to a point, but I was still getting an allergic response if I was exposed to the allergens for a prolonged period. I also noticed that when I got really excited or anxious, I could also induce asthmatic breathing symptoms. These would have been the times I was hyperventilating without being aware of it.

There is a beautiful simplicity about the Buteyko Method. The main practice of Buteyko Breathing involves quiet nose breathing, both in and out through the nose, into the abdomen, so quietly that you can't hear your breath. This is interspersed with pauses between the breaths whilst the breathing is slowed. Surely if it was that simple, why hadn't I been doing it all along? What I noticed though was that when I was in the presence of animals, I was more likely to mouth breathe and start breathing higher in my chest. Even talking excitedly I would gasp in more air between breaths, which dysregulated my breathing. Those subconscious reactions were now conscious.

I decided to put the method to the test. I went to a family party which included coming in contact with a cat. I decided to do everything I knew that would bring on the asthma. I had a sugary drink, I ate party food, crisps and cake and overate at my evening meal. This of course was all in the interest of scientific understanding! Having a full stomach always makes diaphragm breathing more difficult because the full stomach underneath the diaphragm offers more resistance, so breathing tends to occur higher up in our chest, which can initiate the stress response. If the body is already tired and the system is under additional strain, the exhaustion will present itself as a wheeze, in those susceptible.

By the time evening came, I was wheezing away, my chest tight and restricted. Even on returning home I was still struggling with my breathing. I read the Buteyko exercises which involved quiet nose breathing for twenty minutes, with a relaxed *pause* at the end of the out-breath, every minute. I found myself a comfortable position, lying back slightly reclined with my head supported, so that my neck muscles could let go with my abdomen soft and relaxed and not compressed.

Mindfulness and Breathing

The first thing that I noticed was that as soon as the tight-chested feeling occurred, I would automatically switch from nose breathing to mouth breathing. I had no idea I became a mouth breather whilst I was wheezing to try to get as much air in and out as I could. I also noticed I was struggling quite hard against the tension in my chest, trying to get my ribcage to rise and fall against the apparent restriction. My first step was to enable my tummy to be relaxed enough that I could bypass chest breathing so that my chest remained completely still. Placing one hand on my chest and one on my abdomen helped me to focus the movement lower down. I had to trust that I would get enough air.

It was reassuring to know that the aim of Buteyko Breathing is to become comfortable with the feeling of a little bit of air hunger. Using self-hypnosis, I let go and softened my whole body and sunk into the semi-recumbent position allowing my whole body to relax. I imagined letting go of any unnecessary nervous tension in my chest as I let the core of my chest and shoulders relax, as I had done during my hypnosis sessions.

I let my chest stay completely still and noticed with relaxed abdominal muscles how little effort was needed when I was just using the rise and fall of my tummy to breathe in and out. Rather than try to overcome the tension in my chest, I was breathing underneath the tension, into my abdomen. I pictured the breathing going behind my lungs and down into my belly with its rise and fall.

The aim was to breathe without making the wheezing sound as quietly and slowly as possible. I couldn't even feel the breath on the back of my finger under my nostrils, although I was still wheezing. I tried to make my breathing as quiet as I could, but it didn't seem possible. Suddenly I realised that if I used the ujjayi breathing, I could breathe without wheezing, even though it wasn't silent breathing. After one minute of ujjayi breathing (Chapter Five), I could only pause for two seconds at the end of my out-breath before I felt the first desire to breathe. The next breath in after the pause had to be gentle and relaxed. After every minute of yogic ujjayi breathing, I paused at the end of the out-breath for as long as comfortable without tensing.

Ujjayi breathing involves slightly constricting the glottis at the back of the throat and imagining the breath coming in and out through the front of the throat, whilst offering a steady constant pressure to breathe out from the abdominal muscles. Imagine you are making a *Hhaaaa* sound as you would breathe on glass, but with your mouth closed. I didn't know it at the time, but one study showed that the ujjayi breathing can help improve breathing receptors in the lungs which can help with cardiac and respiratory symptoms.[188] I paused again for a couple of seconds at the end of another minute of ujjayi breathing. At the end of the second minute of ujjayi breathing, I paused at the end of the out-breath for about two seconds. I undertook another minute of ujjayi breathing.

The Breakthrough

For the third pause, I used a technique which I have subsequently described to people as the *sink and drop*. It involves bringing your attention to the centre of your chest and then just allowing the front of your chest to sink and imagine your head dropping into the centre of your chest, allowing it to soften and melt, causing any residual tension to release and the mind to rest. Bring your awareness to this area as it softens and relaxes, imagine a warm sensation beginning to expand and open outwards through the chest, spreading through the whole body, as the tension dissipates outwards.

As I sank and dropped into the centre of my chest, it enabled my whole body to relax. It felt as though time stood still in the silence as I expanded my awareness outwards. It was in this moment that everything I had learnt came together. Instantaneously my lungs and chest fully released. The wheeze had entirely gone. It was like flicking a switch. The release that occurred sent a wave of elation through my body. I felt completely at home in my body.

In that third pause, the self-hypnosis relaxation enabled me to relax through the desire to breathe in straight away, like surrendering a fight. This allowed my mind to come to rest, as though in the early stages of falling asleep. When an asthma attack occurs, usually the drive to breathe is significantly heightened with no pause between each breath.

Using the ujjayi breathing means that you can breathe without making a wheezing sound and enables you to return to your breathing after the pause, feeling more relaxed with the small feeling of air hunger, letting go of the panic.

After the third minute of ujjayi breathing and the sink and drop pause, I remained breathing through my nose and into my abdomen, the chest tightness and the wheeze in my lungs had entirely gone. I was able to breathe normally rather than using the ujjayi breath. I immediately remembered my time on the couch seven years previously, where I had felt like I was drowning and I surrendered to the feeling of not being able to breathe, feeling like I was about to die. In the moment that I let go, I must have paused my breathing for long enough for all the airways to dilate and open up. I was excited to realise that I could now repeat the experience consciously. I had found a way of recreating the experience, on my own. The fear had gone.

As I lay resting on my bed breathing with ease, I knew this was something I had to share with the millions of people who suffered from asthma who could all benefit from using this method to relearn their breathing behaviour. More than that, there were countless other people who were hyperventilating with stress and were suffering from stress-related health conditions, who could learn to breathe more effectively and improve their health significantly.

I was so excited by the discovery that I undertook advanced Buteyko training and became a registered Buteyko practitioner with the Buteyko Breathing Association. I also studied breathing biofeedback, known as capnography, which measures carbon dioxide levels on the out-breath to help re-educate a more effective breathing pattern. It is wonderful to be able to share with others how to use this method so that you can also learn to breathe with ease.

STEPS TO MASTERY—Week Five—The Sink and Drop

If you have asthmatic breathing, try using the ujjayi breath to enable you to breathe without wheezing and use mini pauses with the sink and drop technique to enable a warmth to spread through your chest. In order to prevent the wheeze happening in the first place, keep up the healthy living and also add the breathing practice three times a day for four weeks, described in the following chapters.

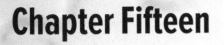

Chapter Fifteen

Retraining Your Breathing

The perfect man breathes as if he is not breathing.

Lao Tzu

A Soft Pause

Through Buteyko's work and my own experience, I had discovered a great way of overcoming an asthma attack. Not only can the method described in the previous chapter stop an attack, if you practise the Buteyko exercises daily it changes your breathing habits over a longer period of time to reduce the frequency of attacks. Even coming into contact with previous triggers, because you have addressed the underlying hyperventilation, your body may have a greater tolerance, helping to reduce symptoms and in some cases clear the breathing issues altogether. The first and most important thing to remember is to breathe in and out through your nose. In addition to this, you can sit and practise a twenty-minute slow-breathing exercise three times a day, including five control pauses. Please *do not* practise the breath pauses if you have any of the following conditions:

- Arterial aneurysm
- Haemorrhagic stroke
- Thrombosis
- Current cancer treatment
- Recent heart attack within twelve weeks
- Brain tumour
- Uncontrolled hypertension (high blood pressure)
- History of serious cardiac rhythm disorder (unless pacemaker fitted)
- Severe renal failure (includes dialysis)
- Uncontrolled hyperthyroidism
- Sickle cell disease
- Acute schizophrenia
- Chronic Obstructive Pulmonary Disease (COPD) with cor pulmonale
- Pregnancy (first trimester)

If you have any of the following conditions *you may* be able to do a reduced version of the Buteyko Method but *only under supervi*sion of a Buteyko instructor. Please *do not* attempt these techniques on your own:

- Diabetes, especially insulin controlled
- Mild / controlled hypertension
- Thyroid disease
- Angina / previous heart attack
- Epilepsy
- Past history of schizophrenia
- Reduced kidney function
- Pregnancy (second and third trimester)

The exercises could lead to changes in your endocrine and nervous system that would need monitoring by your GP.

Practice Makes New Habits

The more you practise, the faster the changes can happen. Your control pause is used to measure progress. From a normal size in-breath, your control pause is the length you can comfortably pause your breath from the end of the out-breath to the next in-breath, without needing any recovery time. Don't try to pause for too long. It is a good idea to take your pulse before and after a session to see if it has reduced or increased. If you have been holding for too long, your pulse is likely to have increased. Ideally, with the relaxed breathing, your pulse should slow with the exercises. Take it easy, you need to be able to recover your slow breathing immediately without any further tension being created.

At the end of your out-breath, you can hold your nose gently during your control pause to prevent you having to tense to hold your out-breath. When you feel your first desire to breathe in, simply let go of your nose and take a normal breath in. You should be able to regain your breathing immediately without gasping or breathing faster. The desire to breathe could be felt as the first push or tensing of your diaphragm. It could also be a feeling in your tummy, chest or throat. The aim of daily practice is to lengthen the time you can comfortably pause at the end of your out-breath. Find ways of relaxing into the tensing with the drive to breathe, towards the end of your pause.

Unless you have any contraindications (see the list above), you can assess how well regulated your breathing is. Take a normal-sized breath in and out, then at the end of your out-breath, with your mouth closed, hold the end of your nose, and time the length of your control pause from the end of your out-breath until your next in-breath. How many seconds can you comfortably manage without needing recovery time afterwards?

If you have a control pause under ten seconds, you would definitely benefit from breathing retraining exercises as there is likely to be significant hyperventilation happening. If you have a pause of between 10-20 seconds you are likely to have moderate dysfunctional breathing. If you want to be out of the asthmatic or reactive spectrum, ideally you would have a control pause of between 35-45 seconds. There is no benefit to pausing for longer than 60 seconds.

Nose Breathing

Nose breathing is vitally important. Not only does it filter and warm the air so that particles of dust do not irritate the breathing passages, as mentioned in Part One, it also produces nitric oxide.[189] This was discovered to be a potent vasodilator to blood vessels by three US scientists in 1998 who won the *Nobel prize for Physiology or Medicine*.[190] Pharmaceuticals have since been produced to improve male sexual potency through the release of nitric oxide in the body. Nitric oxide causes blood vessels to open to enable greater blood flow. Nose breathing is vitally important for many aspects of our health.

Utilising nose breathing, we are enhancing the release of nitric oxide which opens up the capillaries, enhancing blood flow and oxygen uptake in the lungs. It also aids gut motility in the digestive tract. Nose breathing also helps to spiral the air into a vortex to enable smooth laminar flow into the lungs, with minimal turbulence. Overbreathing or hyperventilation is significantly reduced by nose breathing.

Slow Breathing

Buteyko became aware that when people were chronically ill, they over breathe, known as chronic hyperventilation. Many people may think about hyperventilation as someone in the midst of great panic or an anxiety attack. The old trick of breathing into a brown paper bag to slow down the panic and raise the CO_2 levels uses a similar understanding of breathing physiology to the Buteyko Method. There are similarities to 7-11 breathing; counting in for seven and out for eleven with the breath, to reduce anxiety.

Hyperventilation doesn't have to be at the same level as a panic attack to start causing problems. If your breathing rate is subtly increased without your awareness over an extended period of time, your stress levels will be raised by the breathing; it triggers your limbic system to respond as though there is a stressful situation triggering a fight-or-flight response. How many breaths do you take every minute? Set a stopwatch and just count each breath in and out as one. How many breaths did you take?

Although on average people take around twelve to fifteen breaths per minute, some may breathe more. You are aiming to eventually be comfortable with six breaths per minute at rest. It isn't always possible to jump straight to this. Often you need to slow the breathing down gradually. If you find slowing your breathing rate down really difficult, as long as you don't have any neck pain or problems with dizziness, you could look up gently as you breathe in for the count of four and look down as you breathe out for the count of six, to slow the breathing down. This is one of the preparation exercises, but I have used it during breathing retraining sessions for longer when people have found it difficult to slow down. Incorporating the movement with the breathing can help you to relax into a slower breathing rhythm. Don't tip your head too far back, be gentle with your neck.

A breathing rate of six breaths per minute could be in for five and out for five seconds or breathing in for four and out for six. I often think of breathing in for four seconds, out for four seconds and having a relaxed pause at the end of the out-breath for two seconds, where I wait for my body to naturally breathe the next breath in. This makes the breathing more relaxed. Over time with practice, you can gradually slow the breathing down. Maybe begin with having an out-breath just one second longer than your in-breath and then gradually extend each breath in and out.

What Happens at Night?

It is easy enough to keep the mouth closed during the day, but anything could happen during the night. Your subconscious comes out to play during the night, which means that if you are experiencing a stressful dream, you could easily be hyperventilating or mouth breathing. Many people, including myself, have found an improvement in their energy levels and health through taping the mouth closed at night with microporous tape to maintain night-time nose breathing. Use one-inch breathable tape and fold over a tab at each end for easy removal. This should never be done if you have had alcohol, feel nauseous or have taken sleeping tablets.

Nose Clearing

Remember to perform your nip and nod exercises, described in Chapter One and demonstrated on the video before your breathing retraining practice. You can also hold your nose and blow at the end of your out-breath. Repeated nose blowing irritates the mucous membranes and can keep them overstimulated. Never underestimate the importance of dietary change in reducing mucus production too. If excess mucus is a problem, you will need to take steps to find which foods are potentially aggravating this, which you can review in Chapter Seven.

The Method—Week One

First, make sure there are no distractions. Getting into a habit of finding a time and place where you will be undisturbed is a great help. Start by sitting comfortably with your back supported, feet on the floor and hands resting on your lap. Place one had on your chest and one on your abdomen and become aware of where the breathing movement is occurring and whether you are nose or mouth breathing.

Having done your nose-clearing exercises, begin by checking your control pause. It is good to make a note of what your control pause is first thing on waking as it can indicate your progress. It is usually lower first thing but will often improve during the day. It will also be lower after eating so you may want to do your practice before a meal, but it is also good to have relaxation time after eating. It is better to do the exercise than miss it, even if you have eaten. Give yourself room to breathe having had a meal. Leave some space for your breath. It is called a *pause* rather than a *hold* because holding is associated with tension. A control pause requires your body to soften. The control pause will increase quite quickly with practice.

Just like filling a glass with water, breathing should happen from your abdomen upwards, as silently as possible. Begin your first of three daily practice sessions, which last around fifteen to twenty minutes. Silently and slowly, breathe in and out through your nose into your abdomen. Every minute or two measure your control pause and see how long you can comfortably pause and record it in the practice diary. During your breathing exercises, you can perform five control pauses with a couple of minutes of relaxed breathing in between each one. You should always be able to recover within the first breath. If you feel like you want to breathe more rapidly after your pause to regain air, you have paused for too long. Take it steady. You don't need to push yourself, it will come naturally with practice. Try and relax with the feeling of a little bit of air hunger.

Notice what you have to do in your body to lengthen the pause whilst maintaining relaxation through your chest and whole body. I have found in practice that people who have a basic understanding of self-hypnosis master the breathing exercises faster.

Between the pauses breathe in and out through your nose, using your diaphragm and aim to reduce the speed and eventually the volume of each breath.

STEPS TO MASTERY— Weeks Five to Eight

Week One of Breathing Retraining

Make space in your day to do your breathing exercises three times a day. You can do mini pauses throughout the day whenever you feel stressed, to aid relaxation. This means breathing out and relaxing as you pause, and then waiting for your body to want to take the next breath in.

On an evening get used to taping your mouth closed for one hour whilst listening to music or relaxing.

Take a twenty-minute walk each day with nose breathing. This helps to raise your CO_2 levels so that your body starts to become used to having a slightly higher level of carbon dioxide, within healthy limits. If you get breathless, stop, regain your nose breathing and then start walking again. Try breathing down into your abdomen and lower back as you breathe, rather than high up in the chest. Whilst exercising you will likely need to take deeper breaths and faster too, but try to keep your breathing easy and breathe from the bottom upwards.

Week Two of Breathing Retraining

In the second week, you can continue to do the three sessions of daily practice, but you replace the third and fourth control pauses with two extended pauses. The extended pause is a normal control pause, but when you would normally take your breath in you try to extend the pause for five to ten seconds more. You can either tap your chest or rock from side to side to help distract yourself from the feeling of air hunger. Try to regain your relaxed breathing within the first couple of breaths.

Begin by measuring your control pause. Start your relaxed breathing, slowing it down for two minutes followed by a breath pause. Repeat this a second time followed by a second breath pause. Repeat the relaxed breathing two more times with two extended pauses in between. Then relax for a minute at the end before taking your finishing breath pause. See how much you have managed to increase your control pause at the end.

Week Three - Reduced Breathing

In your third week, not only do you try to slow your breathing down, but you also try to reduce the volume of your breathing too. You still add in the extended pause, but you may want to give yourself two or three normal-sized breaths before your extended pause and then return to reduced breathing afterwards.

If you are walking comfortably with nose breathing and have practised this for a couple of weeks, you can commence the steps exercise.

Steps Exercise - Week Three or Earlier

Your breathing isn't going to be as quiet or slow whilst you are walking. Think about breathing from the bottom of your abdomen upwards. After you have mastered nose breathing whilst walking, walk for a minute then pause and return to another minute of breathing through your nose. To measure your control pause time you can count the number of steps you take during your pause, from the end of your out-breath until your next in-breath. Repeat this up to ten times. It should take a maximum of two breaths to completely recover your relaxed breathing; otherwise, you have paused for too long.

If you can't walk, then sitting in a chair and lifting some small weights up and down will help give you some exercise. Once your breath pause has raised to around twenty seconds or more, you could include cycling and counting your pedal revolutions. Wear a helmet, high visibility jacket and lights for your protection.

It can take a bit of practice to become comfortable with nose breathing whilst exercising so build up gradually. Some runners even manage to run with nose breathing, but take steps to build up gradually. If you nose breathe without getting breathless, it means you are not exceeding the body's demand for oxygen and you are exercising within your limits. Adding breathing practice to physical exercise will increase your control pause time faster.

Week Four of Retraining - Very Reduced Breathing

In the fourth week of retraining, whilst doing your breathing exercises at rest, try reducing the size of your breaths even more so that you are only taking small sips of air really slowly. By this stage, aim to comfortably reduce your breathing rate to six breaths per minute. When you do very reduced breathing, you can experience something called resetting. This is when it feels like the breath is breathing itself. You don't feel like you are doing anything actively, but your breathing is slow and easy, almost as though you don't have to breathe at all. It can feel like floating on the breath. If you have this experience, congratulations, you are doing great practice.

You might also want to focus on your speaking and practise reading something out loud taking nose breaths between sentences or during a pause. Taking large breaths whilst talking can also dysregulate your breathing patterns. Don't berate yourself if you catch yourself taking large mouth breaths, simply make the changes when you can.

Keep up the taping at night and the steps routine. One of your practice sessions could be the steps exercise. If you have reached a control pause time of twenty-five to thirty seconds, please see your GP for a medication review. Do not attempt to stop steroid medication without GP advice, as rapidly coming off steroid medication can be life-threatening. Please make sure you get the correct support.

Well done for completing all four weeks of breathing retraining. Keep up your awareness of your breath. Daily practice will help to maintain these changes.

Further STEPS TO MASTERY—The Stop Cough

Many people with asthma don't experience the wheeze as much as they do a persistent cough or need to clear their throat. When you cough it further irritates the airways and causes more inflammation which fuels the problem as this causes hyperventilation as you take in 3-5 times more air whilst coughing. The Buteyko Method advocates using a stop cough technique, which involves the four Ss:

1. Smother   3. Stop breathing

2. Swallow   4. Slow breathing

By placing your hand over your mouth, you bring your awareness to the fact that you are not going to cough. Swallowing creates more saliva and aids relaxation of the throat. By pausing to stop breathing for a few seconds, you help to relax the nervous system and then slowing the breathing helps to prevent further irritation.

Trying to resist tickly, nervous coughs sometimes makes them worse and the urge to cough increases. By relaxing the upper abdomen by placing the heel of your hand just were your ribs meet and gently breathing into this area waiting for it to soften and relax often helps. The other thing to do is only cough through the nose with the mouth closed, to minimise the overbreathing so that each breath is reduced. Pausing at the end of the cough whilst relaxing as you would with a mini control pause helps to regain the breathing balance.

If the cough is more productive, only cough if you feel you are going to move a large amount of mucus. In this case, you can *huff*, as though you are breathing on a pane of glass. If you huff a few times before clearing the throat, it prevents repeated heavier coughing.

At night-time coughing can be worse. When you lie on your back, it can cause the mucus from the back of the nose and sinuses to trickle down the back of your throat and irritate the vocal chords, known as post nasal drip. Sleeping on your side and also adopting a diet without mucus forming foods is helpful.

Yawning and Sighing

Yawning and sighing during your breathing practice or during the day are other sneaky ways your body can over breathe. If you do feel a yawn arising, it is best not to clench the jaw to prevent it but to take a slow long in-breath with the mouth closed. Pause at the top of the inhalation to allow the tension to dissipate followed by a long, slow, sustained out-breath through the nose, pausing and softening the chest and jaw at the end of the exhale.

This can often occur if you have unconsciously held your breath in. This happens when people are concentrating on their work or if they are feeling emotional or stressed and trying to hold it all together. Breath holding on the in-breath is not beneficial for improving the breathing health or stress levels as it generally increases tension throughout the body.

Vigorous Exercise

Walking up a hill, you may want to focus on switching from nose breathing to inhaling through the nose and exhaling through the mouth, before switching entirely to mouth breathing. Always think about the smoothness of the breath and focus on allowing the out-breath to be one second longer than the in-breath. Pursed-lip breathing can slow the mouth breathing so that you keep within healthy limits.

If you are running or swimming getting into a smooth rhythmic pattern of breathing with the emphasis on the out-breath and at the very least keeping the in-breath and out-breath of equal length is important. It is possible with practice to even run whilst nose breathing, which can help to prevent exercise-induced asthma. If at any point during your exercise you notice your breathing becoming more laboured, then stop and immediately regain nose breathing to help prevent you exceeding your oxygen demand. Exercising daily will increase the speed at which you progress.

Why do a Daily Practice for a Month?

Breathing is a behaviour, and just like any behaviour it can be retrained; in the case of breathing, with relative ease. Four weeks is a good length of time to create a new habit or behaviour. It is the CO_2 levels which control your breathing rate in the brain. When you have low levels of CO_2, due to hyperventilation, breathing rate decreases, in some cases to nothing during sleep, causing sleep apnoea.[191] Small increases in CO_2 cause large increases in breathing rate.[192] This means as we exercise we will naturally breathe more rapidly to blow out the extra CO_2.

One theory of how our breathing behaviour is reprogrammed is by changing the tolerance of your brainstem to a higher level of CO_2, whilst resetting your drive to breathe by becoming comfortable (relaxing the nervous system) with the feeling of a little bit of air hunger. This phenomenon is known as resetting. By doing the daily practice over a month our habitual breathing rate, rhythm and how we breathe can be reprogrammed for greater health. This enables the slower, more relaxed nose breathing to eventually become an unconscious habit.

When you exercise your muscle cells produce CO_2 as a waste product. It is the CO_2 which will trigger the red blood cells to let go of the oxygen they picked up in the lungs as you breathed in. This is a highly intelligent system, meaning the oxygen is released only where the demand is highest.

In the long term, having a daily meditative practice for ten to twenty minutes is helpful to keep yourself well. Maintain your nose breathing continually. You may find your night-time breathing automatically becomes nose breathing. If you have eaten late or had a heavy meal or under more stress, you could always tape your mouth. I have taped during the night when in the mountains, at altitude, to enable my breathing to adapt to the low oxygen level faster or if I have had a cold or been particularly stressed.

An Intelligent Response

Naturopathic principles have always suggested that all the reactions in our body are the most intelligent response it can produce, given the current circumstances. This is sometimes hard to believe when we are gasping for breath. However, understanding the mechanism as to why this happens enables us to find a way to change the breathing behaviour appropriately before it creates an adaptive response with unpleasant symptoms.

Why does the body constrict the airways and create more mucus when hyperventilation occurs? When breathing too rapidly the body blows out more carbon dioxide, meaning less oxygen is released into the tissues. As it is the carbon dioxide that stimulates oxygen delivery from the red blood cells into the tissues, less oxygen is delivered when CO_2 is reduced by overbreathing. As hyperventilation disturbs the balance of carbon dioxide and oxygen, constricting the airways is the most intelligent response—slowing down the excess breathing to raise CO_2 to enable better oxygenation. If we fight the constriction, then further tension builds up.

Blood vessels in the body can also constrict as a way of reducing blood flow to raise the CO_2 levels. Carbon dioxide works as a potent vasodilator.[193] This means that as you slow your breathing, blood vessels can open and this can help to drop blood pressure. By breathing too much, it can actually cause a reduction in the oxygen delivered to your body.[194] That is why trying to out-breathe an asthma attack never works. If you have been breathing too much, you simply need to slow things down.

This process is based on the principles of the Bohr effect. The Bohr effect states that when you have higher levels of acid or CO_2 (carbonic acid) in your body, then oxygen will be more readily released from the red blood cells. When there is a lower level of acidity or carbon dioxide, the oxygen stays attached to the red blood cells and doesn't get released into the surrounding tissues. Slowing the breathing down allows more CO_2 to build in your body and provide better oxygenation to the tissues. By relaxing with the feeling of a little bit of air hunger rather than panicking, it will also produce a relaxation response in the autonomic nervous system so your body can let go of emotional tension more easily.

If you chronically overbreathe, the body will create some kind of symptom. In the case of asthma, the narrowing of the airways is the reaction to low-grade hyperventilation. If you look at this as an intelligent response to the overbreathing, you can see how the body is trying against difficult odds to maintain homeostasis and balance. However, if you look at symptoms separate from the whole picture, we see just unpleasant effects that we would want to suppress.

However, as these symptoms are an intelligent response, unless we treat the cause of the overbreathing, the suppression of symptoms alone can cause a worsening of the condition. Sometimes the cause of overbreathing is just a habit that has occurred without conscious awareness. In other cases, it will happen in relation to emotional stresses or digestive stress and reduced fitness, which need to be addressed to help improve breathing health in the long run.

What Can You Affect with Your Breathing?

Breathing helps to regulate many different systems in your body, from your oxygen and CO_2 levels, fight-or-flight activity, to your acid and alkali levels. It can indirectly affect histamine levels, electrolyte (mineral) balance, digestive processes and blood sugar. By regulating and slowing down your breathing, it is possible to have more stable blood sugar. Your mood can become more stable and digestion can be more effective. If histamine levels are lower, inflammation is lower. For reducing allergic reactions having lower histamine levels is great news. Having lower histamine can reduce symptoms of joint inflammation and aches and pains. Most disease processes have some component of inflammation associated with them. Even cardiovascular disease is related to inflammation in the walls of the arteries. As excess sugar gets converted into fat, if your blood sugar is more stable, alongside a healthy diet, there will be less fatty plaque deposition in the arteries.

As the body constricts blood vessels during hyperventilation to raise CO_2, this makes the heart beat harder to overcome the resistance in the narrower vessels, increasing blood pressure. Raised blood pressure has been linked with hyperventilation and studies have shown slow breathing helps reduce blood pressure in many people.[195]

STEPS TO MASTERY—Weeks Five to Eight—Practice Makes New Habits

Record your progress in the weekly diary sheet.

Always measure your pulse before and after your Buteyko exercise set. If you have paused for too long, it will stress your system. Your heart rate should be the same or lower at the end of your exercise set. If your heart rate has increased, reduce the length of your control pause time and increase it more gradually.

Remember, resources (including the Nijmegen Questionnaire) can be downloaded when you register your book.

Chapter Sixteen

Developing Breath Work

In the end, the treasure of life is missed by those who hold on

and gained by those who let go.

Lao Tzu

Buteyko and Allergies

Buteyko believed that if you could raise your breath pause to 35-45 seconds that you would be out of the allergic spectrum. The next time I visited my Dad's house, even in the presence of the cat, I was able to maintain my nose breathing. My breathing stayed relaxed with gentle, quiet breathing into my abdomen, even after eating. I had to be very mindful of keeping my mouth closed to nose breathe. The more I experienced good breathing, the easier it was to relax.

People who experience asthma tend to have a lower tolerance to maintaining nose breathing under pressure. Old memories of previous experiences can increase anxiety, causing a switch from nose to mouth breathing. It is interesting to note that when I was around the cat, my memory of the breathing difficulties caused me to feel a little anxious around the cat, which immediately caused me to feel like I wanted to open my mouth in a stress response. It is easy to see how our breathing and stress can be so intrinsically linked. The more I practised the relaxed nose breathing, the easier it became.

When you slow down your breathing rate, breathing efficiently into the abdomen, you enable greater oxygenation of your body and reduce the stress response. You may actually start to feel more relaxed. Any time you notice any anxiety around your breathing creeping in, do a mini control pause of a few seconds at the end of your out-breath and soften your chest and solar plexus and imagine it opening outwards in the pause.

When your body is less stressed your body eliminates waste more effectively, it absorbs nutrients better and maintains higher levels of health. The immune system is not as overloaded with waste to eliminate. By practising the simple breathing exercises on a regular basis, three times a day over the course of a month, the breathing then starts to automatically become slower and more relaxed. The brainstem can reset to being comfortable with a new CO_2 level, which is more natural for your health.

The Healing Crisis

In this period of resetting, your body has to bring a new balance to all the different systems in the body. Initially, there can be a further healing crisis, where your body throws out waste products more rapidly to help this resetting process. This can involve greater mucus production, increased kidney elimination or even diarrhoea, a sore throat, headache or skin rash or a cold. Sometimes even old memories or emotions come to the surface. As you allow this process of letting go, on the other side of this eliminatory effort, your health usually improves and breathing becomes easier. With some dedication, using the exercises you can make a significant improvement to your health quite rapidly. This process can be supported by fasting or eating fresh, living foods and resting.

Floating on the Breath

If there is a great deal of tension associated with the breath, it can be enormously helpful to remember to focus on your favourite place of relaxation whilst you do your exercise rather than focusing too much on the breath. Sometimes when we focus too much attention on something we actually create tension. By imagining yourself in your favourite place of relaxation, your breathing will automatically slow down. As you begin to reduce the volume and the rate at which you breathe, still breathing into the abdomen, you will find that you can begin to float on your breath. By this, I mean that you can watch yourself breathe your breath, rather than you actively breathing yourself. By pausing at the end of each out-breath for a second or two and waiting for your body to naturally take the next in-breath, it becomes easier to let go of the breath and let go of control.

Children and Buteyko

Children will not have the patience to sit still doing relaxed breathing. For adults and children over seven you can make it more interesting using the *steps* exercise. Walk with nose breathing for a minute. At the end of a minute from the end of an out-breath count how many footsteps you can take before your next in-breath. The number of steps becomes your control pause measure. Continue walking for another minute whilst nose breathing. After a minute perform another control pause and count how many steps you take. You can repeat this with ten control pauses each interspersed with one minute of nose breathing as one of your daily exercise sets. You must be able to recover your breathing within two nose breaths. Read the information about the steps exercise in Chapter Fifteen.

If it is difficult to walk breathing through the nose, then start by standing, relaxing your body and breathing into your tummy with your shoulders dropped. When you pause, march up and down on the spot and see how many steps you can do on the spot. This is a useful addition if you can't get out of the house. If you get really good at the exercises, you can try doing star jumps in the pause. The idea is to be able to recover the breathing so that you come back to slow abdominal breathing with the shoulders dropped and relaxed within a couple of nose breaths.

If you are practising indoors, children are encouraged to hold their nose, to prevent them from cheating and taking a sneaky breath in during the pause. This exercise is suitable for children from around the age of seven. There are basic relaxation breathing exercises for younger children.

Case Studies

Rose was in her early thirties and successfully used the Buteyko Method along with some minor dietary changes, cutting out wheat and dairy, to come off her asthma medication, which she had been on since being a university student. Even during the winter months, she didn't have a problem with her usual cold, where previously the asthma would be exacerbated. She remained mindful of her nose breathing and keeping her breathing slow, steady and relaxed. Two years on she has given birth naturally to a beautiful baby boy and is still asthma free, without medication.

Natalie was in her mid-forties when came to see me, having just been discharged from hospital with severe asthma. Arriving at the clinic with a pulse over 100 at rest, and gasping for breath, having just walked 25 metres from the car park, I was concerned. She had been given oral steroid medication whilst in hospital. Her lips were blue, and when I checked her oxygen saturation level, it was 85%. Oxygen saturation should ideally be above 95%.

We went through a very gentle Buteyko set together. And I was pleased to see that during the session, using a pulse oximeter, her blood oxygen saturation was rising to a more normal value after the mini pauses. Natalie practised three times a day with only a small control pause so as not to stress her heart rate. She returned a week later, her lips no longer blue, her heart rate down to around 85 at rest and her oxygen saturation was 92%. I was amazed by the difference. She continued her exercises and went on to make a good recovery and has been delighted that she can walk again without getting breathless. She had been steadily deteriorating before she started her breathing exercises.

It is inspiring to see such determination and dedication in people to make a difference to their health. You can too. It is important to value yourself enough to make the changes. Many people might think it is the easy path to keep doing what you are doing and just take medication when the results of modern living result in illness. Having ill health is never an easy path in the long run.

I strongly believe that suppression is not the answer. In the end, we trade one condition for another until our body cannot compensate any further. The only real solution to long-lasting health is to provide the right rest, sunlight, nutrition, emotional support, exercise and breathing re-education where necessary to help us move forwards. Illness tends to come with an exhausted nervous system and inadequate nutrition, so giving your body time to heal and recover is very necessary. If you have taken steroid medication, it takes time to rebuild your strength. Dedicate a whole year of your life to improving your health. Once you have a healthy routine, it will be easier to continue.

Eye-Roll Technique

Both the Buteyko Method and hypnosis use an eye-roll technique. In Buteyko practice, the eye-roll is helpful to lengthen the breath pause. The eyes are linked with a reflex reaction to slow the heart rate and breathing as we roll our eyes upwards. This is what happens when we fall asleep. By reducing the fight-or-flight response, it helps to reduce the drive to breathe and switches into the more relaxed part of the nervous system. In hypnotherapy, the eye-roll is used to induce a trance state, which immediately switches us out of our stress response and into relaxation. This is not to be performed with contact lenses or if you have an eye condition.

When you focus on an area of tension within you, as you breathe into the tension, look down into that area and imagine scooping the tension up and out of your head with your *vision* as you breathe out. During the pause soften your body and expand your awareness. It is possible to release areas of shock which may have been held for many years. Once you let go your body can restore health. Adding in the ujjayi breathing can have a more powerful effect of releasing the tension when combined with an eye-roll and breath pause.

The Birth of Dynamic Breath Release

During my stay in Australia, I learnt how to breathe into my abdominal tension and breathe it out through the top of my head. Propped up in bed I combined a deep breath with the eye-roll technique I had learnt during my hypnotherapy training, inducing a rapid relaxation in my system. Once home I began to use this whilst doing cranial osteopathy on patients to breathe the tension I felt out of the body, and also encouraged people to use it themselves. It worked incredibly well. Adding in the ujjayi breath made it more powerful.

Whenever an emotional issue arises for me, I recognise the polarity that I am experiencing. At the other end of the magnet is the opposite polarity. Somewhere between the two is the neutral point. Once I have breathed through the emotional tension that has arisen, I make sure I feel fully connected to the earth under my feet, so that I am grounded. I then imagine a funnel in the top of my head and imagine the opposite polarity pouring in through the crown of my head and down into my body, neutralising the old issue. For example, if you have a fear of rejection, you would identify the tension in your body, breathe into it for a couple of minutes as you acknowledge how it has tried to protect you, and then at the end of the out-breath, scoop the tension up and look up and send it out through the top of your head. The opposite of rejection might be self-acceptance. You could then imagine breathing this in through the crown of your head and into the previous places of tension, allowing your body to soften and release into this in the next pause as it spreads through your body. You may even breathe in some new inner resources that can enable you to move forwards with greater ease, imagining a future where you feel free.

Sometimes you have to give yourself the time and space to be able to relax and heal. Giving yourself a well-earned holiday where you can truly let go and have access to fresh produce whilst you are there, will give your body the opportunity to heal. It is your tissue intelligence that heals, not you. You can't will a fractured bone to mend, but you can have it set in the correct position and stop yourself from worrying about whether it will mend or not. Trust your lungs can heal too and relax your ribcage. Give yourself permission to let go.

Dynamic Breath Release in Practice

As I developed my Buteyko practice, it was really interesting to notice that the breath pause with relaxation and mindfulness could be used to brilliant effect to help release old, stored trauma. One client had suffered a traumatic delivery of her first child and had been suffering from lower back pain since. She was also suffering from asthma.

Although conventional osteopathy brought some release to her lower back, the tension kept returning. We also added in Buteyko training to help overcome the asthma she experienced, combining osteopathy to help release the overly contracted neck and shoulder muscles which had become shortened and tense from upper chest breathing over many years. During one of the sessions, we focused on using the ujjayi breath to breathe down into the lower abdomen. I asked her to breathe into her uterus and on the out-breath, use a control pause whilst rolling her eyes up towards the top of the head where she softened the lower abdominal area. Similar to the release from my asthma attack, to our amazement in that moment, Jane noticed that her back pain had immediately released and has been clear for several years since.

When she stood up, I checked her pelvic alignment. Her body had come back to normal positioning. We were both stunned by the rapid change. Osteopathy is wonderful for releasing tension, but if the gentle stretching and realignment are combined with releasing emotional shock and trauma with breathing, there is a more lasting effect which appears to restore greater health. Rather than just treating the symptomatic area it addresses the cause.

The change was lasting. The following week during her Buteyko practice Jane also reported feeling warm hands and feet. She had previously been diagnosed with Raynaud's syndrome which causes fingers or toes to often become white with cold and has no known medical cause. She was finding a way to improve her circulation. By relaxing the fight-or-flight nerves, which would cause blood vessel constriction, she was allowing the condition to reverse naturally.

Breathing effectively supports the inherent natural healing of your body, and can kick-start a process which may have been chronic for years. Combining the traditional Buteyko Method with Dynamic Breath Release to shift emotional holding is a powerful tool for recovering parts of us that have been through trauma. By being aware of what memories might be surfacing for you whilst breathing, you can simply relax your body as you breathe through them and reintegrate those lost parts of you that became separated by the trauma, letting go of the old emotional tension in the pause. The recovery of lost parts can lead to your recovery.

Using Dynamic Breath Release with Emotional Eating

Your perception is often heightened when you take time to breathe and meditate. New insights can occur once old emotional tensions have been released. During a breathing workshop, Louise looked at her relationship with food and overeating which left her feeling *fed-up*. She recognised that her independent streak had led her to find comfort in food rather than with people and she had a habit of stuffing her emotions down with food and then criticising herself harshly, which led to further guilt and limiting behaviours.

During her Dynamic Breath Release session, Louise recognised that she had mistakenly believed that she couldn't ask for help or support—she had to do it all herself. As soon as she recognised this, she made a commitment to herself to ask for help when needed and nurture herself with food. Louise felt greater freedom with what she ate. She had also been in the habit of rushing her eating with a busy schedule. She committed to mindful eating, noticing when she was full and only eating when she was hungry. Louise was able to let go of the food fight.

If overindulgence has happened and you reduce your intake or have a cleansing day the next day, this will support the recovery from the additional strain placed on the system. Make sure you don't criticise yourself harshly for the past choices you have made. Be kind to yourself with your future choices and know that you can ask for help and support. You can become used to feeling so well from eating light, energising foods, that to feel heavy and lethargic is not a comfortable choice to make. It is always important to fill the space that you have cleared with something positive and beneficial in its place. It can be a positive feeling instead of food.

Inner Dialogue with Dynamic Breath Release

Once in a relaxed state, you can speak to parts of your body and ask them what they need. When I asked my lungs what the problem was, I got a real sense that they felt tired from overwork. I too had worked too hard and pushed myself too much. The real underlying issue was a fear of not being loved. I wonder how many times this issue might arise in your life? Do you create all kinds of behaviour to prevent yourself from feeling this fear? Behaviours could range from overwork to over-giving, and even beating ourselves up for not being enough. You may have experienced this. Your willingness to recover the underlying emotion so that it no longer controls your behaviour means that you can finally give yourself space to relax and just be rather than spinning yourself into endless activity. There is a simple solution. You can give the inner child inside you the love you have been looking for externally. In your control pause, soften your heart to unconditional love for you.

Going with the Flow

Ultimately your breathing should not be forced into a particular pattern. In health, we are constantly adapting. Your breathing and breath should be a natural response to your different experiences. You may find that when you have strong emotions in your abdomen that you need to match the power of your emotions with the intensity of your breathing. If you have strong emotions in your chest and heart region, it is necessary to work with this using very gentle nose breathing to find release and expansion of your awareness into the softness of love and tenderness.

With every breath in, you can breathe love into your heart, and with every out-breath, this life force spreads through your whole body and being. When you soften in the space between each breath, you can receive more love, presence, peace of mind and greater freedom.

STEPS TO MASTERY—Week Eight—Using Dynamic Breath Release

By now you should be able to integrate the Dynamic Breath Release, using ujjayi breathing with the breath pause and eye-roll whenever strong emotions surface for you. This will help you to move through emotions more easily. Remember to always breathe into a feeling of inner peace or love to replace whatever you have released with something more supportive for you now. You may find having your story witnessed makes it easier to release emotional tension. The simple breathing practice can also do a lot to reduce the mind chatter and the strain on the nervous system, calming down many of the emotional responses.

Chapter Seventeen

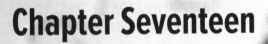

Discovering the Ease

Breath is the bridge which connects life to consciousness, which

unites your body to your thoughts.

Thich Nhat Hanh

The Final Piece of the Jigsaw

Buteyko and Dynamic Breath Release were the final pieces of the jigsaw. It enabled the penny to drop. I could stop the endless searching for solutions to health problems. Every therapy works along similar lines. They all work to reduce the overactivity of a stressed or even exhausted nervous system, to enable your body to do the healing. They all work to help relax the body, which in turn will help to relax the breathing. If you can work with your breath to slow things down, you can work with your body rather than against it.

Initially, osteopathic treatment helped me to release the wheeze, by restoring balance within the nervous system and calming nerve overactivity. During the thoracic adjustments I had paused at the end of the out-breath long enough to let go, reducing the fight-or-flight activity which reduced the breathing rate. This is turn eased the need for congestion. Osteopathy can create space inside you, enabling your body to make the necessary adjustments. I still wanted to find a way of creating that internal space myself without having to rely on treatment.

Learning guided meditation enables you to engage with your emotional field and your non-physical reality, giving you a connection with your energetic system and the breath. Guided meditation can deepen your consciousness by facilitating the release of subconscious fears that can drive your breathing and limiting behaviours. Connecting with your heart essence enables you to release these old issues so that you can find deeper freedom. By clearing these patterns at their roots, the tension dissipates and the body and mind find a new equilibrium, creating more space inside. As the emotional holding lessens, so does the breathing.

The change in nutrition gives your system so many fresh vitamins and minerals to enable the blood to be more effectively buffered so that the breathing doesn't have to do all the work of blowing out excess acid. A low-inflammatory, plant-based, whole-food diet also reduces the inflammatory and mucus forming foods in the body and supports the elimination of waste. Energising yourself with the appropriate nutrition enables your body to have greater reserves to clear the backlog of waste, as clearing this requires energy to produce the transformation. Any belief system can become dogmatic if taken to its extreme. It is important to realise these methods are all tools to allow you to access your authentic self and let go of parts of you that are no longer supportive of your health. Understanding and working with the principles of Nature Cure means that you learn to trust your body's natural healing processes.

Hypnotherapy and mindfulness teach you how to transform limiting beliefs and break habit patterns that can sabotage your best attempts at making changes. Being able to self-hypnotise will make you more mindful of when tensions are creeping in and how to relax the fight-or-flight nervous system when unnecessary nervous tensions arise. It enables peace of mind and automatically causes the breathing to slow down without even focusing on it. As you relax your body, the brainwaves slow down, and your breathing slows too.

The Buteyko Method works so easily to draw everything together. Slowing the overbreathing down is easy when everything else is in place. Even the emotional rollercoaster, overthinking and worrying can lessen when the breathing is slower and no longer feeding into the drama of the unnecessary fight-or-flight response. The mind is then more at rest. Using what you have learnt throughout this book will bring about an understanding of how to use Dynamic Breath Release as a powerful tool to deal with emotional issues as they arise. Rather than resisting them, recognise these past parts of yourself are presenting themselves for healing. It is an empowering way for you to be able to transform yourself. A whole universe of possibility is waiting in the pause at the end of your out-breath.

Slowing your breathing down on its own is powerful. Slowing your breathing down becomes much easier when you take care of yourself as a whole, but waiting for everything to be perfect before you begin never works. Notice the areas of your life that are causing you the greatest stress and work on resolving these issues. Release your fears of the unknown and step into a new reality which enables you to reconnect with the opportunity for better health. There is no one single thing which will bring you out of chronic health into wellness again. If you want the whole of you to be well, you have to take care of your whole life, but start with small changes, and make them consistently. If you build on each small change, before you know it you will be miles away from where you first began and can begin to bring greater ease into your life.

New Beginnings

Having retrained your breathing to be slower and more relaxed, it can simply take care of itself as long as you remain mindful of how you are feeling. If you are stressed or anxious about anything in your life, you may have to be more mindful of calming your breath or resolving the underlying emotion for your breathing to remain easy.

In the early days, it is so important to take things slowly to build your confidence. For example, starting ahead of the hay fever season and, where possible, not exposing yourself to previous allergens whilst retraining the breathing will help to give your system a rest whilst changes are made. Also cutting out foods which your body doesn't tolerate is also an excellent way to enable your immune system to be in peak condition. Your digestive ability will improve with the breathing exercises, however stoking your internal vitality with the best fuel possible enables your health to significantly improve, whatever your condition.

Finding out where the main tensions lie, whether there is a build-up of mechanical tension, emotional tension or physiological strain from digestive issues will help to guide you as to which changes are most important. Finding a way to release the emotional tensions naturally will reduce the fight-or-flight activity. If you slow your breathing down, often emotions don't escalate as much. However, some can grip us significantly. Working with Dynamic Breath Release can be helpful to enable you to reconnect with your true self, beyond the waves of the emotions.

Many different people have used the Buteyko Method to help other conditions such as lowering their blood pressure, releasing tension headaches, some have even found their blood sugar levels improve, or hot flushes decrease with the control pause. On its own, breathing effectively is an immensely powerful transformative tool. The digestive process becomes markedly more efficient with proper breathing, but it isn't an excuse to forget about good nutrition, regular activity or healthy lifestyle choices—these *enhance* the effects of Buteyko practice.

If you are looking for greater energy more consistently, then I can wholeheartedly recommend natural living with mindful breathing. There is no one magic cure-all. There are simply natural, healthy choices, which support your body's innate healing ability. Good health then becomes a choice you make. The healthy choices you make may not mean you live longer, but as long as you make them wholeheartedly, they make the ride along the way more comfortable. At times of challenge, your body needs more care and support. These are the times to be vigilant to take even greater care of yourself and ask for help when needed.

Using a Focused Pause

When your attention is directed externally, tension can arise. You have no control over your external reality, only how you respond to it internally. When you have your awareness focused on the inside, if you are resisting what you are experiencing, you will notice where the tension of your emotional response arises. Rather than fighting the thought, you can simply focus on softening the tension in your body related to the thought. If you then breathe into the area and on the out-breath, pause and soften the area, it can help the tension to release. Bring your attention back to where you have some control. Always remember the main control you have is your choice to either hold on or let go. Letting go is more comfortable in the long run. This is where we find freedom.

I had spent my whole life wondering why chronic diseases maintained themselves. The adaptations your body's intelligence brings about are the best it can do with the current resources it has. Giving your body greater resources with improved breathing, rest, nutrition, movement and love it is possible to overcome mountains.

Having seen the results of working with the mindfulness meditation group, I had realised the power of guided meditation but realised it was important that people could practise their exercises in the comfort of their own home. I also wanted to make this work accessible to everyone, so I started a project to help people rediscover their own innate power to transform their health.

Giving yourself twenty minutes a day just to be with your breath is the greatest gift you can give yourself. It requires dedication, but you are worth every moment. It is your recharge time to live your life to its fullest potential.

Natural Health

Can you imagine the benefits breathing with ease has on all your internal organs as you fully let go and relax through the core of your body and being? Imagine how it feels to work with your body rather than against it. It creates a greater feeling of harmony and ease. Begin to find the peace you often strive for, by effortlessly working with your body and breath. To simply rest deeply is a healing experience in itself. Just take a moment right now to indulge yourself. Feel the very centre of your chest melt with your out-breath. And begin to feel a warm, pleasant sensation begin to spread from your chest, down into your fingers, and down into your toes. As you do so, softening through your whole body, imagine yourself in your favourite place of relaxation, where you feel completely at peace, and unconditionally loved.

If you are suffering from a chronic health condition, depending on your level of vitality and determination, it is possible to improve your health naturally and make a change. Work on it as though it is a project rather than identifying yourself with the condition and a label. It is worth taking positive action before your body starts screaming at you with symptoms to embrace healthy living.

The great natural healers all believed there were no diseases, only obstructions to your natural bodily functioning. These obstructions could be at the physical, physiological, nutritional or emotional level. When we remove the blockage, then health can be restored. The strength of the symptoms is proportional to the level of vitality which is blocked. If you have a strong symptom, you have a huge amount of vitality or emotional charge which is being blocked by tension and holding patterns. The block might be a limiting belief, or it may be a repetitive strain injury creating tension, or it might be a diet which produces too many waste products which overload your tissues or ferments in your gut and stops you breathing deeply.

If you can transform your frustration into determination, anything is possible, but it was never in the striving that I found what I was looking for. By doing the work to prepare the ground to create a change, it enables you to function more effectively meaning you can fall into a healthy relaxation so much more easily. When you release the blockage, you release the potential energy to step forwards into freedom.

There may be aspects of your health that are beyond your capability to change. These aspects offer us opportunities to focus our lives in a unique direction. The first step towards healing is often finding acceptance of where you are and learning to unconditionally love your imperfect self, for what you may believe to be your weakness can become your greatest strength. Without the asthma and allergies my drive to learn and discover healing methods that would support myself and others would not have been as strong. It was always a gift in disguise.

Natural healing isn't for the faint-hearted. It takes courage and trust and often a step into becoming comfortable with the unknown. You hold the whole universe within ourselves. Once you have created space in your pause, you can choose what you fill this space with. Every time I pause and soften my chest now, I allow in the feeling of space and then breathe in unconditional love and gratitude for life. It feels like the tingles of joy and excitement as you look up into the magical, starry, vastness of space. As you breathe out this wave of unconditional love and gratitude can spread through your entire being.

Clearing the internal struggles with the breath as they come along doesn't get rid of life's challenges but empowers you to be able to let them go with ease and create the life of your dreams. It seems to bring a greater feeling of lightness. The emotional dramas become fewer and when your breathing is slower your emotions are more settled. It's like tuning into a smoother frequency. You can find release from your mind-made prisons. The door is open; you are free to fully embody your radiant self and your own unconditional love, for you.

Yes, challenges still arise, and I am by no means perfect. Perfection is not the aim. The intention is to reconnect with *you*, to unconditionally love all of you and live an authentic life. Failure is inevitable, as many of our habitual patterns are deeply ingrained, and whilst we begin to commit to a new way of life, old habits will surface. We often learn more from our failures, which of course means there are none. Success comes when we bounce back undeterred from setbacks with self-compassion. Find acceptance for where you are and remember the darkest hour is just before dawn. Your challenges can give you a greater desire for something new as long as you are prepared to turn and face that direction.

I would never have believed that it was by breathing less that I could improve my health. Combining this with a deep trust in life, and living in accordance with the laws of nature and eating food in its natural state, gives us a natural way through life. Through understanding and embracing natural healing, you can begin transforming your health.

The tendency is there if you push your body to revert to old patterns, just as when you don't vacuum your carpets, dirt soon accumulates. Now you know a new way of approaching health which can be applied to improving overall health, not just breathing difficulties. Natural healing is not a treatment for a condition; it is a way of life which promotes health. The acute symptoms are the body trying to have that extra spring clean, and the chronic is simply the best adaptation your body could make to the challenges you found yourself in. In this moment there are new opportunities and new choices to be made.

I spent years trying to escape myself, and make myself somehow different, or running away from what I was feeling or experiencing. When I finally discovered the answer had been there all along, inside of me, when I stopped fighting myself and surrendered, it felt like coming home. In your pause, you can reconnect with unconditional love for yourself, just as you are. This joyful feeling of coming home to yourself is always here, waiting and ready for the moment when you let go. Value yourself enough to honour your health and well-being consistently.

Every challenge becomes an invitation to access a deeper aspect of yourself. I spent too many years looking for healing and love on the outside. It is in the space between each and every breath you take. You only have to pause to reconnect with it. My understanding of healing is to bring wholeness or oneness to mind, body and spirit. The breath unites the whole of your being. It is the link between the inside and the outside of us and the connection between the physical and non-physical aspects of us. Like the air that surrounds us and unites and holds us all, we find a connection to all of life through the breath. Through the breath, we connect to this moment and reconnect with our oneness. In the pause, you become the bridge between heaven and earth.

The ease is in the space between the breaths. When you find the courage to let go and trust, it creates the space to enable you to start living the life of your dreams. Use your new-found vitality to embrace life with joy and happiness and love. You too can breathe with ease.

This is just the beginning....

ACCESS THE REEFERENCES ONLINE

(no need to register)

www.breathewithease.co.uk/references

ACKNOWLEDGEMENTS

To my parents, Michael and Annette, for supporting me with love throughout my life and through my osteopathic training and my siblings, Rowland, Mel and Benjamin and family who have been my greatest teachers. To my grandfather, for inspiring me to become an osteopath and naturopath and launch my healing journey and my dear departed Nanna, without whom I wouldn't have set upon a lifelong journey to rediscover health.

My teachers, in particular the osteopathic teachers who really inspired me; John Wernham, Quentin Shaw, Sarah Boswall Wheeler, Howard Beardmore, Tim Sparrow, Miriam Elkan, John Parsons, Anna Reeve, Gez Lamb, Peter Blagrave and Renzo Molinari, and all those at the Institute of Classical Osteopathy and the European School of Osteopathy. My naturopathic and Nature Cure teachers Leslie Harrison, Peter Fenton, James Johnson and John Fielder. Brandon Bays of *The Journey*. Vernon Frost, metaphysical teacher, guide and mentor for over a decade. The London College of Clinical Hypnosis teachers. The Buteyko Breathing Association teachers; Janet Brindley, Catherine Moffat, Gillian Austin and Kathryn Godfrey. Brigitte Martin Powell and Doug Sawyer who created Avalon Institute of Rebirthing (AIR).

The ISRN and Nature Cure Trust for supporting the writing of this book and related projects and giving me a platform to teach this work.

I am grateful for those that helped catalyse an awakening, particularly Barry Male, who not only taught me how to abdominal breathe but held a space for my first breakthrough. A huge thanks to Annett Jowett, my mother, who enabled the creation of York Natural Health, and to all those who work alongside me, I deeply appreciate your support.

To Richard Hagen and Martyn Pentecost of DotDotDot, my publishers.

To my friends, past and present, who have encouraged me, believed in me and given me love.

To all the patients and clients I have worked with over the years, who have inspired me with their courage and determination and revealed what is possible with natural healing.

ABOUT THE AUTHOR

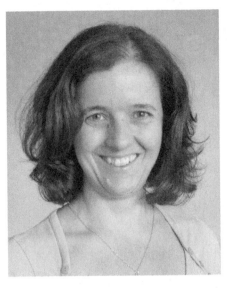

Alison Waring is creator of the *Breathe with Ease Method* and *Dynamic Breath Release*. She is the clinic director of York Natural Health. With more than twenty years of training and practice in osteopathy, naturopathy, Journey Therapy, clinical hypnotherapy, Buteyko Breathing, rebirthing and yoga, Alison offers a holistic, natural approach to all areas of health care.

After struggling for many years with her own asthma challenges, in 2011 she overcame an allergic asthma attack, naturally, in three minutes. She did this using her own Dynamic Breath Release technique. Wanting thousands more to enjoy the freedom she now enjoys led her to further refine and develop Dynamic Breath Release. This approach allows emotional challenges to be released effectively, through the breath.

When the underlying causes of dis-ease have been addressed, the body's natural healing systems can bring true healing from the inside. The Breathe with Ease Method provides the stepping stones to support your natural healing from within.

Alison offers breathing workshops, one-to-one consultancy and is a speaker on natural health, particularly asthma and other breathing challenges. As chairman of the Nature Cure Trust charity and secretary to the ISRN, the oldest naturopathic register in the UK, Alison supports the professional community and promotes understanding of natural health in all its dimensions.

www.breathewithease.co.uk

www.yorknaturalhealth.co.uk

Other dot dot dot publishing Titles

The Little Book of Holistic Accounting

Emma J Perry

ISBN–978-1-907282-81-2

For those stuck in a job or path that is stifling. How to balance the books of your body, mind, heart and soul.

Unconscious Incarceration

Gethin Jones

ISBN– 978-1-907282-86-7

For those who are stuck in repeating patterns of self-destructive behaviour. How to recognise the patterns, change your mindset and take action.